THE COMPLETE 2024 FOODS LISTS FOR DIABETES

Unlocking the Power of Nutrient-Rich Foods - Explore a Variety of 300+ Low Glycemic Load Options in this Comprehensive Guide

Dr. Vivian Greene

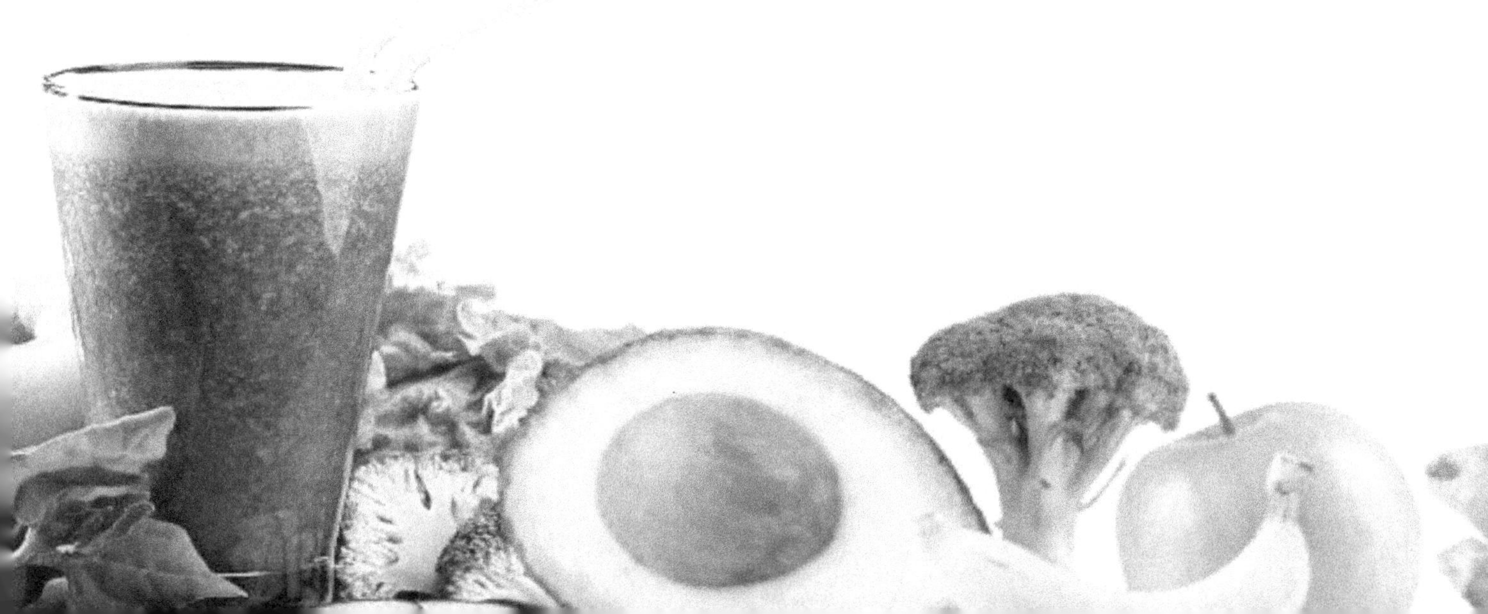

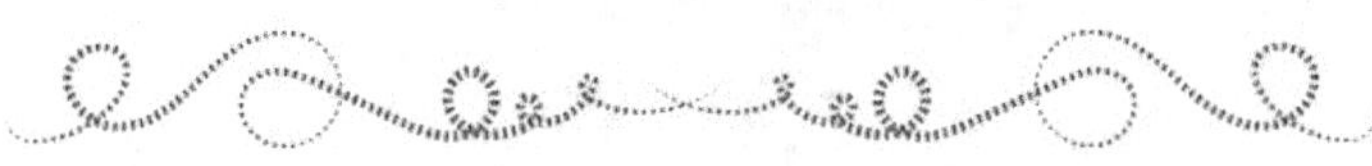

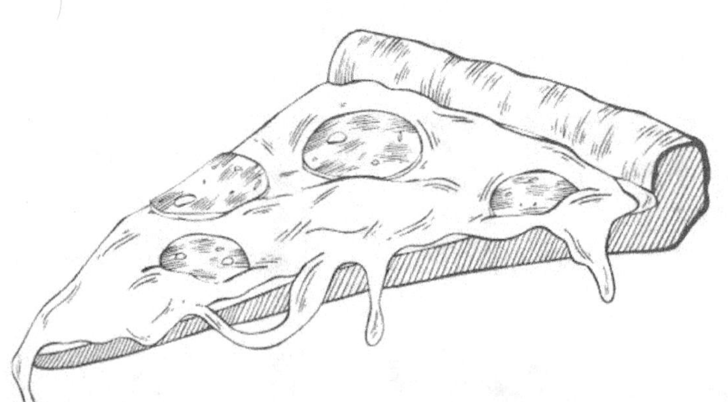

Copyright © 2024 VIVIAN GREENE

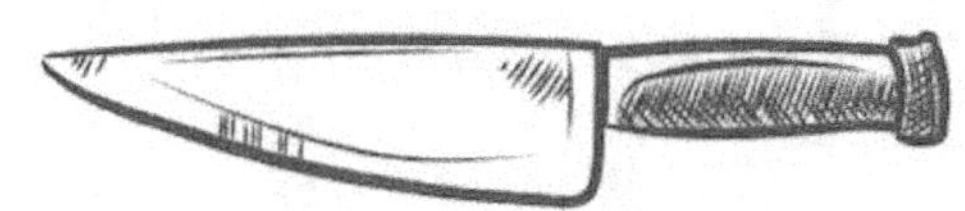

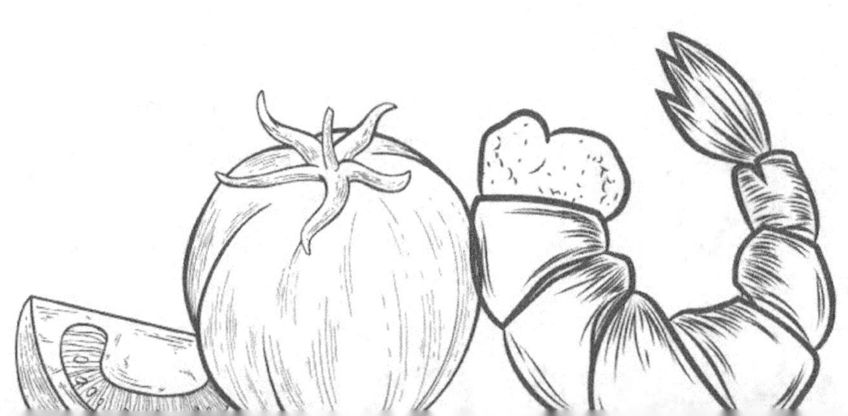

Table of Content

Foreword

As we navigate the complexities of managing diabetes, the role of nutrition emerges as a cornerstone in achieving optimal health outcomes. In this comprehensive guide, readers are equipped with a treasure trove of knowledge and practical insights into crafting balanced, diabetes-friendly meals. With a focus on nutrient-rich choices and mindful meal planning, this book serves as a beacon of guidance for individuals seeking to take control of their health journey. Written by experts in the field of nutrition and diabetes management, this invaluable resource is sure to empower and inspire readers on their path to wellness.

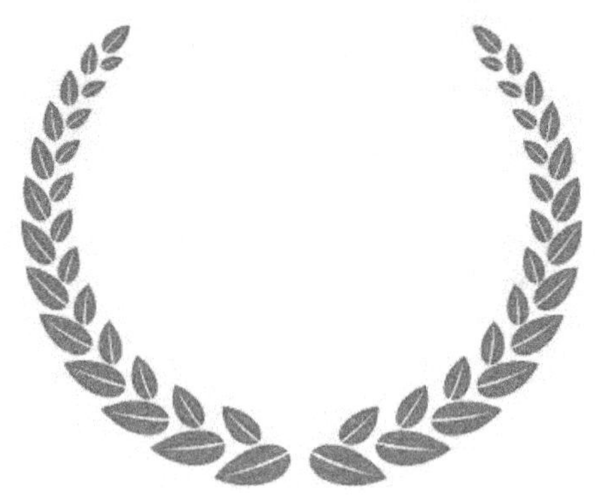

Dedication

This book is dedicated to all those who face the daily challenges of managing diabetes with courage, resilience, and determination. Your unwavering commitment to prioritizing your health and well-being serves as a constant source of inspiration for us all. May this book serve as a beacon of hope and empowerment on your journey towards optimal health and vitality.

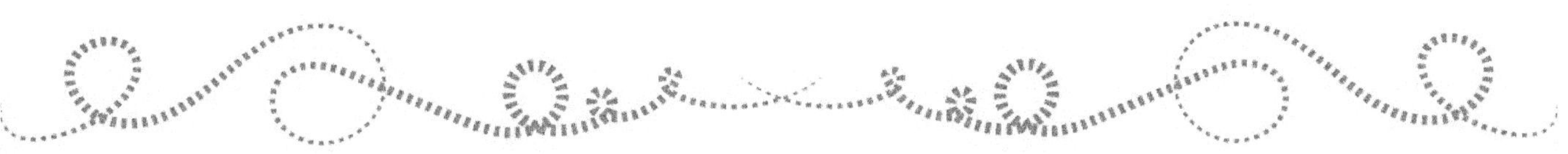

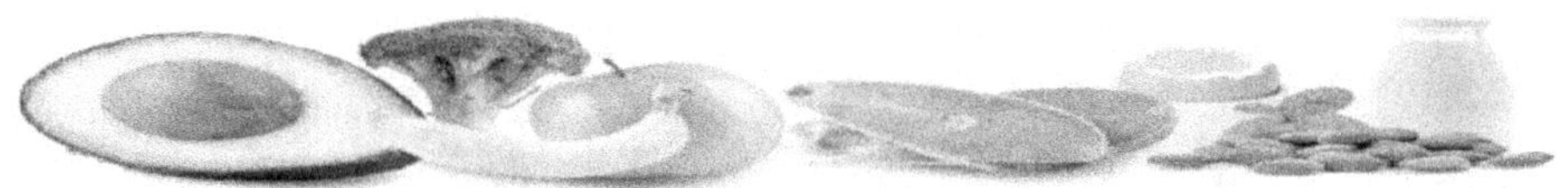

Introduction

With great pleasure, I provide this indispensable tool to assist people in their quest for efficient diabetes care.

It may be difficult to navigate the complexity of diabetes in today's fast-paced society, when convenience often takes precedence over nutrition. But with the correct information and resources, we can take control of our health and make decisions that will improve our quality of life.

This book is a monument to the empowering and educating power of knowledge, not just a collection of recipes. These sections provide lists of more than 300 nutrient-dense foods that have been carefully chosen for their low glycemic load and ability to promote stable blood sugar levels. However, this book is more than just a list of meals; it's a thorough guide that provides useful perspectives, professional guidance, and detailed methods for incorporating these foods into your everyday routine.

The main goals of this book are to help readers understand the idea of diabetic meal lists and provide them the resources they need to choose their diets wisely. People with diabetes may take proactive measures to properly manage their condition by learning about the concepts of glycemic index (GI) and glycemic load (GL) and become adept at navigating the wide variety of dietary alternatives available.

This book is for you whether you have had diabetes for years or are just receiving a diagnosis. I really hope that reading these pages will provide you a better knowledge of the role diet plays in managing diabetes as well as give you the confidence to take charge of your health and adopt a lifestyle that encourages energy and well-being.

Are you prepared to start this life-changing adventure? Together, let's unleash the potential of nutrient-dense foods and open the door to a better, more healthful future.

Understanding the Significance of Diet in Diabetes Management

A balanced diet may also help with weight control, which is another important aspect of managing diabetes. Maintaining a healthy weight via eating is crucial for general health and well-being since excess weight may develop insulin resistance and raise the risk of cardiovascular disease.

Beyond regulating blood sugar and helping people lose weight, a healthy diet may also have a favorable impact on blood pressure, cholesterol, and general vitality. People with diabetes may improve their general health and lower their risk of long-term issues by making nutrient-rich meals a priority and adopting a balanced eating pattern.

A balanced diet has many physiological advantages, but it may also have significant psychological ones, such as empowering people and giving them a feeling of control over their health. People who have faith in their abilities to make educated food decisions are more likely to follow their treatment regimen and take an active role in their care.

Realizing the transformational potential of food as medicine is ultimately key to comprehending the role of diet in diabetes control. People with diabetes may maximize their health results, enhance their quality of life, and flourish despite their disease by adopting a nutrient-dense eating pattern that is customized for them.

The Impact of Nutrient-Rich Foods on Blood Glucose Levels

The connection between meals and blood glucose levels is crucial when it comes to managing diabetes. Foods high in nutrients are essential for controlling these levels, which has a significant effect on the general health and well-being of diabetics. Foods high in vitamins, minerals, fiber, and other critical elements are known as nutrient-rich foods. These meals have special properties that may help regulate blood glucose levels. Nutrient-rich meals provide a more steady and slow release of glucose into the circulation than processed diets heavy in refined sugars and carbs, which may result in sudden increases in blood sugar levels.

The fiber content of many nutrient-rich meals is a major element in this stabilizing effect. Fruits, vegetables, whole grains, legumes, and nuts all contain fiber, which slows down the breakdown and absorption of carbs to help avoid sudden spikes in blood sugar. Furthermore, fiber increases feelings of satiety and fullness, which may aid in weight management and lower the likelihood of overeating for those with diabetes.

These meals are beneficial to heart health and lower the risk of cardiovascular problems linked to diabetes since they are often low in cholesterol and saturated fats. Furthermore, the vitamins, minerals, and antioxidants included in nutrient-dense meals enhance immune system performance, facilitate tissue regeneration, and reduce inflammation—all of which are vital factors to take into account for those who are managing a chronic illness like diabetes.

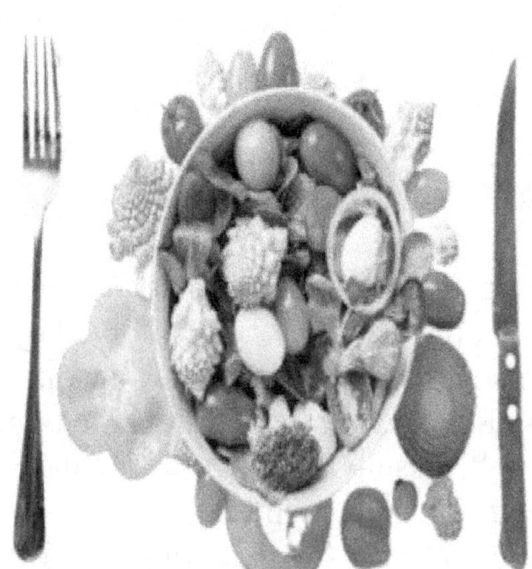

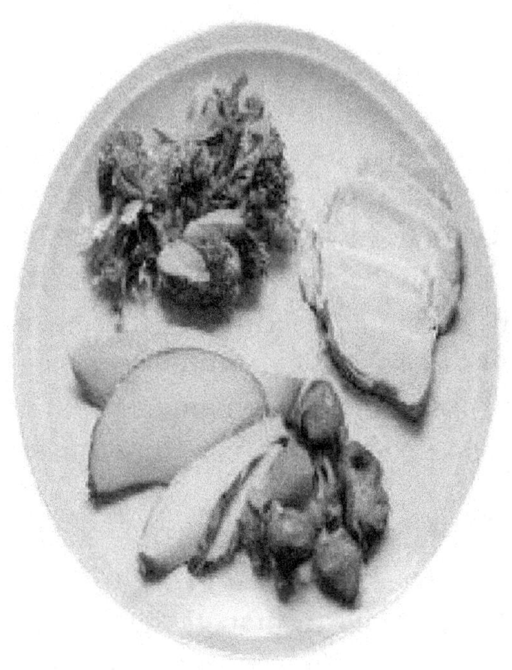

Essentially, nutrient-dense meals have a far greater effect on blood glucose levels than just counting carbohydrates. People with diabetes may make use of the nutritional potential of whole grains, fruits, vegetables, lean meats, and healthy fats to improve blood sugar regulation, improve general health, and prosper on their path to maximum well-being.

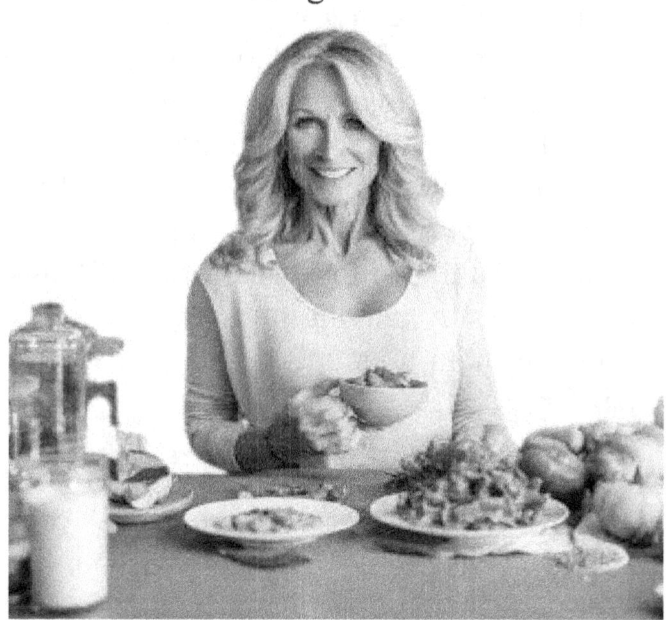

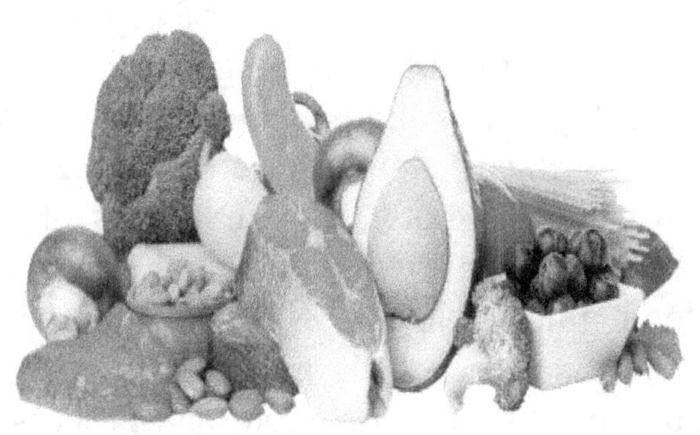

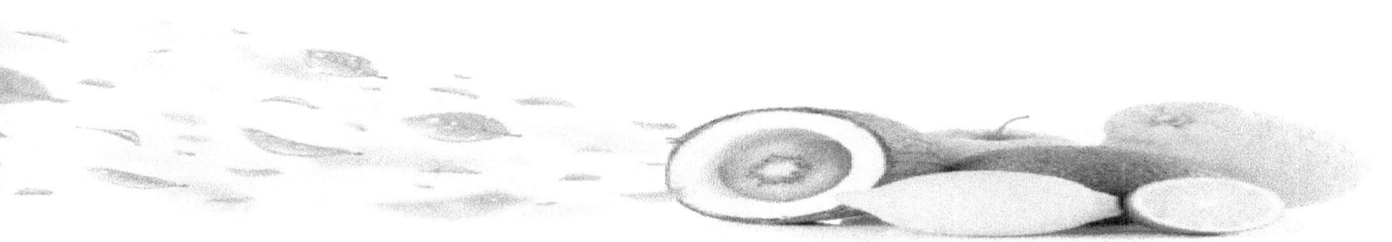

OVERVIEW OF THE COMPREHENSIVE GUIDE

Greetings and welcome to the extensive guide " The 2024 Complete Foods Lists for Diabetes: Unlocking the Power of Nutrient-Rich Foods - Explore a Variety of 300+ Low Glycemic Load Options in this Comprehensive Guide" We will present you with a quick rundown of what's included in the pages of this priceless resource in this part.

This manual is intended to act as a road map for anybody looking to improve their diabetes control by making knowledgeable food decisions. This book is designed to meet you where you are on your path to improved health, regardless of how long you have had diabetes or how recently you were diagnosed.

Over 300 carefully chosen low-glycemic-load meals that support stable blood sugar levels and enhance general well-being are the foundation of this extensive guide. To help you make informed nutritional choices, each food item is accompanied by comprehensive information on its glycemic index (GI), glycemic load (GL), and net carbohydrate content.

This book provides a plethora of useful information and professional guidance to assist you in navigating the difficulties of managing your diabetes, in addition to comprehensive meal lists.

All of the chapters are jam-packed with useful tips and success techniques, ranging from knowing the greatest and worst foods for diabetes to learning the science-backed glycemic index (GI) and glycemic load (GL) diet concepts.

In addition, this book offers customized suggestions and comprehensive meal planning instructions to assist you in preparing well-balanced, diabetes-friendly meals that satisfy your unique dietary requirements and tastes. This book has all the information you need to improve your A1C and blood glucose levels, hone your diabetes management techniques, or acquire essential nutritional knowledge to avert complications from diabetes.

To put it briefly, "Unlocking the Power of Nutrient-Rich Foods" is a comprehensive resource that goes beyond a book and gives you the tools you need to take charge of your health and change the way you manage your diabetes. Are you prepared to start this life-changing adventure? Together, let's explore and harness the potential of nutrient-dense foods.

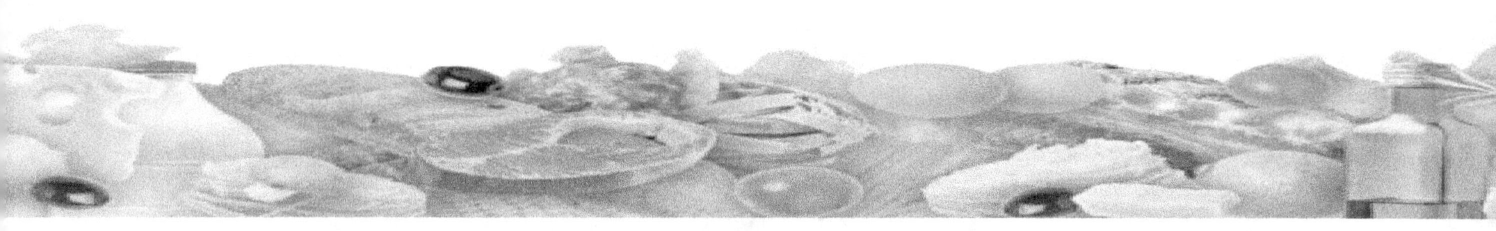

The Science of Glycemic Index (GI) and Glycemic Load (GL)

The science of glycemic index (GI) and glycemic load (GL) must be understood by anybody hoping to control their blood sugar levels, especially those who have diabetes. These two ideas are useful for evaluating how diets high in carbohydrates alter blood glucose levels and provide information on how various foods might influence the body's metabolic processes.

The glycogen index (GI) is a system of numbers that ranks carbohydrates according to how much they may increase blood sugar levels when compared to a reference item, usually white bread or pure glucose, which is given a value of 100. Foods with low GI values (below 55) are digested and absorbed more slowly, resulting in a steady and continuous release of glucose into the circulation. Conversely, foods with high GI values (above 70) are swiftly digested and absorbed, causing a sudden surge in blood sugar levels.

GL, on the other hand, provides a more thorough evaluation of a food's effect on blood sugar levels by accounting for both the amount and quality of carbs in a serving. It is computed by taking the food's GI, multiplying it by the quantity of carbohydrates it contains, and then dividing the result by 100.

While foods with a low GL have a more moderate influence on blood glucose levels, those with a high GL may produce considerable swings in blood sugar levels, especially if ingested in large amounts.

People may reduce their risk of hyperglycemia and hypoglycemia and promote stable blood sugar levels by making educated dietary decisions by knowing the fundamentals of GI and GL. For instance, choosing meals like whole grains, legumes, fruits, and non-starchy vegetables that have low GI and GL will help sustain consistent energy levels and lessen the chance of blood sugar spikes and crashes.

adding a range of low GI and GL items to meals and snacks will help improve glycemic control over time, which will lower the risk of complications from diabetes and improve hemoglobin A1C levels. Additionally, emphasizing nutrient-dense, low GI and GL meals may help maintain general health and well-being by offering vital antioxidants, vitamins, and minerals that support healthy physiological function and the avoidance of illness.

The terms Glycemic Index (GI) and Glycemic Load (GL) refer to two basic ideas that help explain how various diets impact our blood sugar levels. It is important to comprehend these ideas, particularly for those who are treating diseases like diabetes where controlling blood sugar is critical.

First, let's discuss the Glycemic Index (GI). GI is a technique of classification used to group carbohydrates according to how rapidly they cause blood sugar levels to rise after eating. High GI foods are quickly absorbed and digested, which causes blood sugar levels to rise quickly. On the other hand, meals with a low GI digest and absorb more slowly, which causes blood sugar levels to increase gradually but steadily.

GI is mostly interpreted using a numerical scale, which normally runs from 0 to 100. those that have a GI value of 55 or below are categorized as low GI, those that have a GI value of 56 to 69 as medium GI, and those that have a GI value of 70 or above as high GI. People may lessen the chance of abrupt spikes or falls in their blood sugar levels by selecting meals with a low or moderate GI.

Let's explore Glycemic Load (GL) now. Although the Glycemic Index (GI) offers useful information on how certain meals impact blood sugar levels, the Glycemic Load considers the kind and amount of carbs that are taken. It is computed by taking the food's GI, multiplying it by the number of carbs per serving, and then dividing the result by 100.

This sophisticated method of GL gives a more realistic picture of how a dish affects blood sugar levels since it takes into account both the total quantity of carbs taken and their rate of digestion. those with a high GL have the potential to significantly alter blood sugar levels, particularly when ingested in large amounts; those with a low GL have a less noticeable impact.

People may make educated dietary decisions that support stable blood sugar levels and general health and well-being by knowing the fundamentals of GI and GL. Choosing low-GI and low-GL foods, such as fruits, whole grains, legumes, and non-starchy vegetables, may help control blood sugar levels, enhance glycemic management, and lower the risk of complications from diabetes.

understanding the underlying theories of the Glycemic Index and Glycemic Load enables people to take charge of their health by selecting meals wisely. By applying this understanding to their eating patterns, people may more effectively control their blood sugar levels and create the foundation for a happier, healthier life.

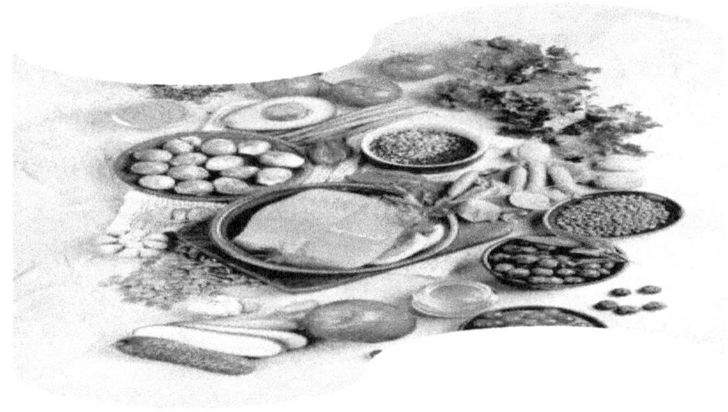

Glycemic load (GL) and the glycemic index (GI) are two important ideas that influence how various meals impact blood sugar levels. Let's examine the workings of these phrases to understand their impact.

Let's start by talking about the Glycemic Index (GI). Foods high in carbohydrates are ranked according to how rapidly their ingestion raises blood sugar levels. High GI foods are quickly absorbed into the circulation after digestion, which causes a sharp rise in blood sugar levels. Conversely, meals with a low GI value are absorbed and digested more slowly, which causes blood sugar levels to rise gradually over time.

Let's now discuss Glycemic Load (GL), which accounts for both the amount and quality of carbs in a meal. Whereas GI just looks at how quickly carbs are absorbed, GL takes into account a food's carbohydrate content as well as how it affects blood sugar levels to provide a more complete picture. While foods with a low GL have a more moderate influence on blood glucose levels, those with a high GL may produce considerable swings in blood sugar levels, particularly if ingested in large amounts.

So how do GI and GL affect the levels of blood sugar? Our blood sugar levels may jump quickly when we eat items high in GI and GL, including sweet snacks or refined carbs like white bread and rice. Insulin, a hormone that aids in transferring glucose from the circulation into cells for use as fuel or storage, is released in response to this abrupt increase. On the other hand, excessive insulin production in reaction to a sharp rise in blood sugar levels may cause a decrease in blood sugar that results in symptoms like hunger, exhaustion, and irritation.

On the other hand, consuming low-GI and low-GL foods such as legumes, fruits, vegetables, and whole grains may support more stable blood sugar levels. Because these meals take longer to digest and absorb, the circulation releases glucose gradually and continuously. Because of this, insulin is released more gradually, which helps to reduce abrupt changes in blood sugar levels and encourages sensations of fullness and continuous energy.

A food's glycemic load (GL) and GI are important factors in determining how it affects blood sugar levels. People may maintain more stable blood sugar levels, decrease their chance of blood sugar spikes and crashes, and improve their general health and well-being by selecting meals with lower GI and GL values.

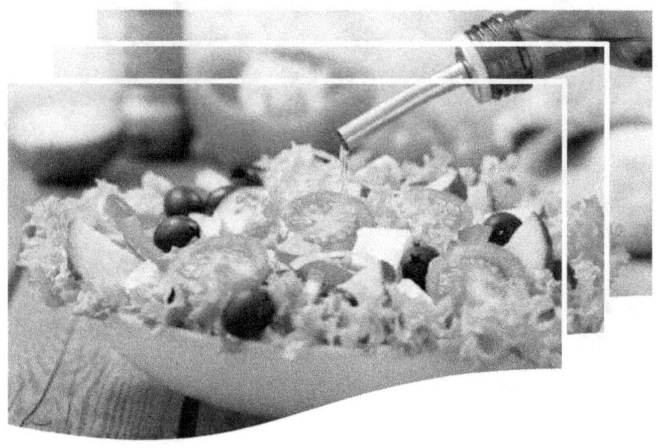

People with diabetes need to maintain a balanced diet since it helps control blood sugar levels, improve general health, and lower the risk of complications from diabetes. A balanced diet provides the body with the necessary nutrients while maintaining stable blood glucose levels. It does this by including a range of foods that are high in nutrients in the right amounts.

Maintaining good blood sugar levels is one of the main objectives of diabetes care. This may be accomplished with a balanced diet that includes low levels of processed foods and refined sugars, as well as complex carbs, lean proteins, healthy fats, and fruits and vegetables high in fiber. Because complex carbs like whole grains and legumes digest more slowly, blood sugar spikes are avoided and glucose is released into the circulation gradually.

A balanced diet not only helps regulate blood sugar levels, but it's also critical for maintaining a healthy weight—something that's especially critical for those with diabetes. Gaining too much weight may aggravate insulin resistance, making it harder to regulate blood sugar levels and raising the risk of problems including cardiovascular disease. People with diabetes may attain and maintain a healthy weight, which lessens the strain on their bodies and improves overall health outcomes, by eating a balanced diet that prioritizes nutrient-dense, low-calorie foods and encourages portion management.

A well-balanced diet offers vital vitamins, minerals, and antioxidants that are critical to general health and wellness. Lean proteins, whole grains, fruits, and vegetables are examples of nutrient-rich diets that are high in beneficial elements that boost immune system function, encourage tissue repair and lower inflammation. People with diabetes who prioritize these items in their diet may boost their immunity, lower their risk of infection, and maintain good physiological performance.

A balanced diet may also lessen the chance of developing diabetes-related problems such as kidney disease, heart disease, stroke, and nerve damage. Diabetes patients may reduce their risk of cardiovascular disease and other chronic illnesses linked to the disease by eating meals low in saturated fats, cholesterol, and salt. The risk of diabetic neuropathy, a frequent consequence of diabetes that may cause numbness, tingling, and discomfort in the limbs, can also be decreased and nerve damage can be prevented by maintaining stable blood sugar levels with a balanced diet.

it should be noted that a balanced diet is crucial for managing diabetes. People with diabetes may successfully manage their disease, enhance overall health outcomes, and lower their risk of complications from diabetes by adhering to a diet that emphasizes nutrient-rich foods, portion management, and moderation. In addition to helping to regulate blood sugar, eating a balanced diet is crucial for fostering long-term health and well-being.

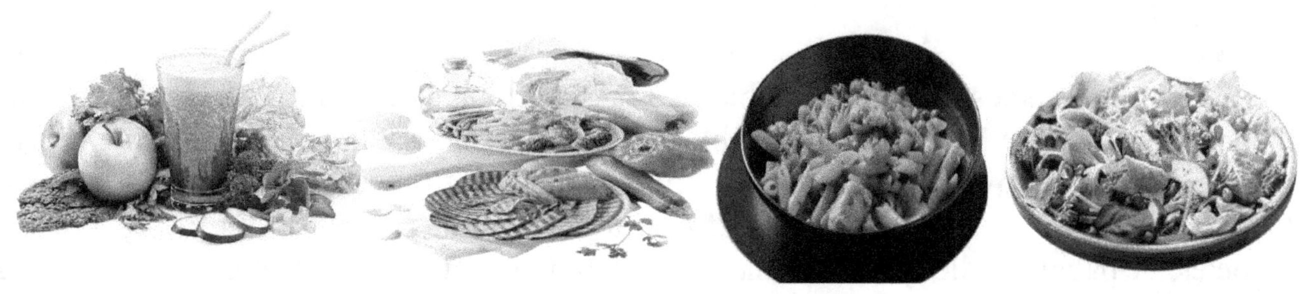

The Power of 300+ Low Glycemic Load Foods

The idea of glycemic load (GL) is important when it comes to managing diabetes. It is an essential tool for everyone trying to efficiently control their blood sugar levels and preserve general health. Low glycemic load foods stand out among the many dietary alternatives available as potent allies in this attempt, providing a host of advantages that may have a good influence on managing diabetes and general well-being.

The capacity of low glycemic load meals to provide a slow and steady increase in blood glucose levels helps to avoid abrupt spikes and crashes that may upset metabolic homeostasis. Low glycemic load meals take longer to digest and absorb than high glycemic load foods, which means that the amount of glucose released into the circulation is more steady and lasts longer.

Because they may help with glycemic management and lower the risk of complications from diabetes, low-glycemic load foods are important to include in one's diet. Choosing these foods may help people control their blood sugar levels, which will enhance their hemoglobin A1C levels and lower their risk of hypo- and hyperglycemia. Low-glycemic meals provide health advantages beyond controlling blood sugar. They often include high concentrations of vital elements that are important for maintaining general health and well-being,including vitamins, minerals, fiber, and antioxidants. People with diabetes may increase their nutritional intake, strengthen their immune systems, and lower their chance of developing chronic illnesses like cardiovascular disease and certain types of cancer by including a range of these nutrient-dense foods in their diets.

The adaptability of low-glycemic load meals opens up many culinary options, which facilitates the maintenance of a satisfying and balanced eating pattern. With so many low-glycemic load alternatives available, it's easy to prepare enticing and fulfilling meals that support diabetes control and advance general health. These options range from whole grains and legumes to fruits, vegetables, lean meats, and healthy fats.

The value of 300+ low-glycemic load foods is found in their capacity to boost general health and well-being for people with diabetes, stabilize blood sugar levels, and improve nutrient intake. By adding these items to their diet, people may take advantage of nutrition's transforming power to control their diabetes more effectively and open the door to a happier, healthier life.

Gaining a comprehensive knowledge of the foods we eat is the first step towards managing diabetes effectively. Here, we explore the long lists of foods that have been carefully curated for people with diabetes, providing a wealth of information to help make educated food choices and achieve optimal health.

Our carefully chosen meal lists provide a wide range of alternatives, each one chosen for its effect on blood sugar levels and overall nutritional content. Every food item, including whole grains, lean meats, fruits, and vegetables, has been assessed to make sure it is suitable for inclusion in a diet that is diabetes-friendly.

The GI and GL of each food item are important factors to take into account while creating these meal lists. We provide people with useful information about how various foods might impact blood sugar levels by classifying foods according to their GI and GL values. This enables people to make decisions that promote stable glycemic management.

Our lists of foods are made to accommodate a range of dietary needs and tastes, so people with diabetes may eat a lot of delectable and filling things. Our meal lists include a wide variety of options to accommodate various dietary requirements and tastes, including vegetarian, vegan, gluten-free, and low-carb diets.

Our lists not only provide a wide variety of meals, but they also include helpful advice on serving suggestions and portion proportions. For people to control their blood sugar levels and calorie consumption, knowing the right portion sizes is crucial. Our comprehensive suggestions help people make informed dietary decisions.

In the end, perusing our comprehensive lists of foods specifically designed for people with diabetes is about enabling people to take charge of their health and well-being by making educated dietary decisions. Through the adoption of a diverse and well-balanced diet abundant in foods high in nutrients, people may enhance their general health, effectively manage their diabetes, and lead more fulfilling lives.

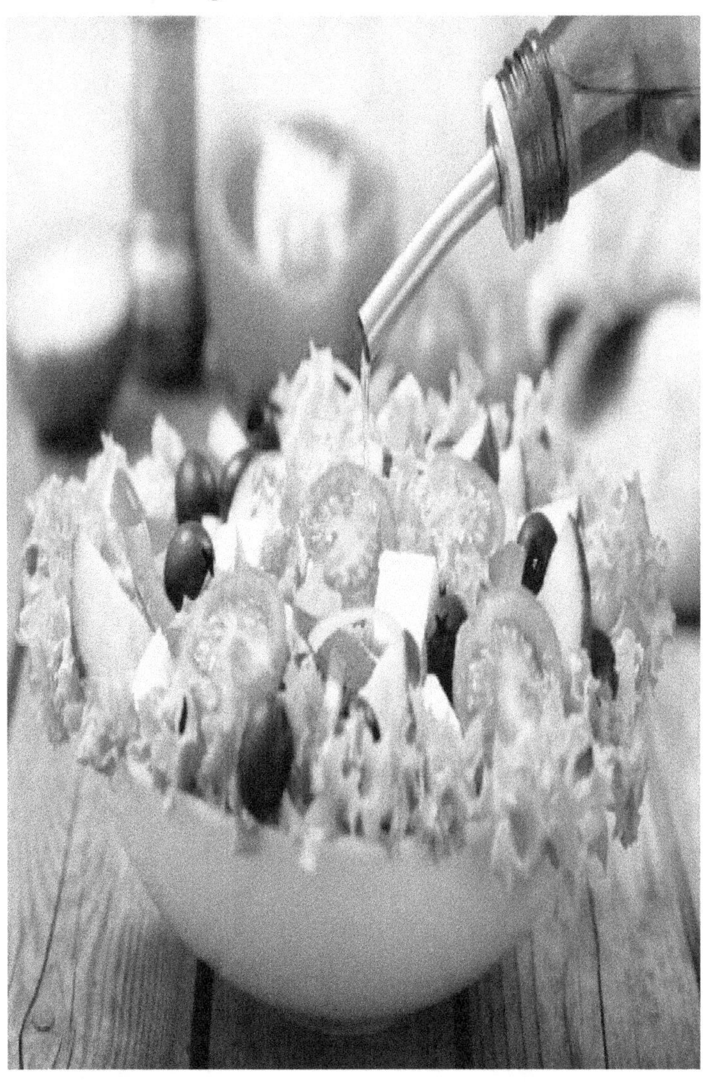

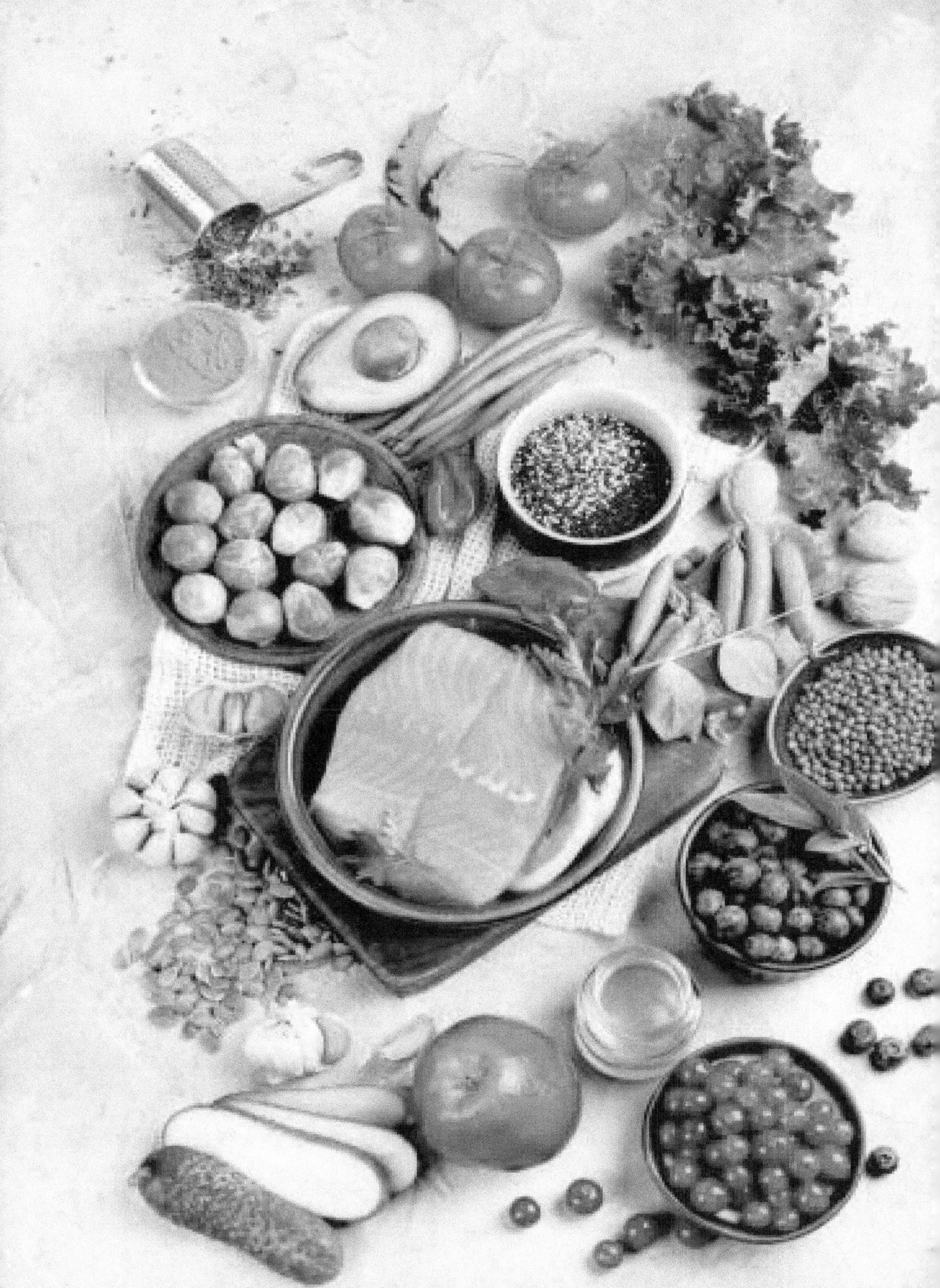

Benefits of Low Glycemic Load Options for Diabetes Management

There are several advantages for people with diabetes who choose meals low in glycemic load (GL). These choices have the potential to be very beneficial in controlling blood sugar levels, enhancing general health, and lowering the likelihood of problem outcomes.

Helping to balance blood sugar levels is one of the main advantages of low glycemic load alternatives. Low Glycemic meals release glucose into the circulation more gradually and sustainably than high Glycemic foods, which may induce fast blood glucose rises followed by crashes. In addition to lowering the risk of hyperglycemia and hypoglycemia and fostering more stable glycemic control over time, this consistent energy source helps avoid abrupt swings in blood sugar levels.

A further important component of managing diabetes is weight control, which is something that low glycemic load alternatives may help with. The high fiber content of many low-GL meals helps people feel satisfied with fewer servings and decreases the chance of overeating by promoting feelings of fullness and satiety. Individuals with diabetes may lower their risk of insulin resistance and enhance insulin sensitivity by adding these items to their diet and maintaining a healthy weight or reaching weight reduction objectives.

In addition, there are other nutritional advantages to low glycemic load foods beyond controlling blood sugar. A large number of these foods are high in vital vitamins, minerals, and antioxidants that promote general health and well-being, making them nutrient-dense. Diabetes sufferers may make sure they are getting the nourishment they need while also lowering their chance of developing chronic illnesses like heart disease, stroke, and certain forms of cancer by selecting low-GL meals such as fruits, vegetables, whole grains, and lean meats.

Accessibility and adaptability are two further benefits of low-glycemic load alternatives. It is simple for people with diabetes to have a balanced and fulfilling diet since these items are widely accessible and can be included in several different meals and snacks. You may include low-GL foods into your regular eating patterns in a variety of ways, such as adding berries to your oatmeal for breakfast, having a salad with grilled chicken and mixed greens for lunch, or having sliced veggies and hummus as an afternoon snack.

For the treatment of diabetes, low glycemic load choices provide clear advantages. These meals provide a comprehensive approach to diabetes treatment, aiding in weight control, regulating blood sugar levels, supplying vital nutrients, and enhancing general health. Individuals with diabetes may improve their quality of life and lower their risk of problems by including a range of low-glycemic alternatives in their diet. This is a proactive approach towards greater health and well-being.

Incorporating Variety for Balanced Nutrition

A balanced diet provides our bodies with a wide range of nutrients that are necessary for optimum health and well-being, not just the fundamental requirements. To make sure we get all the vitamins, minerals, antioxidants, and other vital elements required for maintaining physiological function and avoiding illness, diversity in our diet is critical.

The idea that no one meal can provide our bodies with all the nutrients they need to flourish is one of the cornerstones of nutrition. Every food category has a distinct mix of nutrients to give, so we can make sure we're getting all the nutrients we need by eating a range of foods from various categories.

Fruits and vegetables, for instance, are abundant in vitamins, minerals, and antioxidants that help the immune system, encourage a healthy digestive system, and guard against long-term conditions like cancer and heart disease. Make it a daily goal to include a rainbow of fruits and veggies in your diet. Choose from a range of hues to make sure you're receiving a wide range of nutrients.

Whole grains include complex carbs, fiber, and vital elements like iron and B vitamins. Examples of whole grains are brown rice, quinoa, oats, and whole wheat. You may support digestive health, encourage fullness, and help regulate blood sugar levels by including a variety of whole grains in your meals.

Lean meats, chicken, fish, eggs, tofu, legumes, and nuts are examples of foods high in protein that are necessary for tissue growth and repair, hormone and enzyme synthesis, and muscle maintenance. To make sure you're receiving the full spectrum of amino acids in your diet, try to incorporate a combination of plant- and animal-based protein sources.

Nuts, seeds, avocados, olive oil, and fatty fish are good sources of healthy fats that are essential for hormone synthesis, brain function, and the absorption of fat-soluble vitamins. Including a range of healthful fats in your diet may improve general well-being, cognitive performance, and cardiovascular health.

It's crucial to choose a variety of meals from each food category in addition to making varied selections within each group. To make your meals interesting and pleasurable, try experimenting with new sorts and tastes of fruits and vegetables instead of sticking to the same ones every time.

You may lower your risk of dietary deficiencies, increase general health and energy, and make sure you're getting the nutrients you need by adding diversity to your diet. To achieve balanced nutrition and thrive on your path to maximum health, don't be scared to experiment with different meals and tastes.

Mastering the GI & GL Diabetes Diet

Taking the first step toward taking charge of your health and successfully controlling your blood sugar levels is learning the Glycemic Index (GI) and Glycemic Load (GL) diabetic diet. Through comprehension of the underlying concepts of this method and use of workable techniques, you will be able to make well-informed food decisions that support stable blood glucose levels and improve general health.

Fundamentally, the GI & GL diabetic diet places more emphasis on the kind and amount of carbs eaten than it does on the overall amount. This method allows you to select meals that have the least amount of influence on glycemic response by accounting for the many ways that carbs affect blood sugar levels.

Understanding the GI values of different foods is crucial to mastering the GI & GL diabetic diet. Low GI foods—those with a GI of 55 or less—digest and absorb slowly, raising blood sugar levels gradually and giving you prolonged energy. Whole grains, legumes, non-starchy vegetables, and the majority of fruits are foods that have a low GI. However, meals with a high GI (70 or above) absorb and digest more quickly, which causes blood sugar levels to jump sharply. To lessen their effect on the glycemic response, these items should be eaten in moderation or combination with low GI meals.

Understanding the GL component of the diet requires not only taking into account GI values but also evaluating the total amount of carbohydrates in meals and how that affects blood sugar levels. You may assess a meal or snack's ability to elevate blood sugar levels and make necessary modifications to maintain optimum glycemic control by calculating its GL. Foods having a high GL (20 or more) should be taken in moderation or in conjunction with low GL foods to reduce glycemic swings. Low GL foods are the best options for stabilizing blood sugar levels.

The following are some useful tips for navigating the GI and GL diabetic diet:

Giving priority to whole, minimally processed foods: Processed and refined foods, which often have higher GI and GL values, should be avoided in favor of whole grains, fresh fruits and vegetables, lean meats, and healthy fats.

Meal and snack balance: For stable blood sugar levels and long-lasting energy, try to include a mix of healthy fats, proteins, and carbs in each meal and snack.

Being aware of portion sizes: When eating foods with higher GI and GL values, pay particular attention to portion proportions. To lessen their effect on blood sugar levels, use smaller portions or combine them with meals that have a lower GI.

Trying out different meal combos: To maintain glycemic control while keeping meals engaging and fulfilling, try out various meal combos and recipes that include a range of low GI and GL items.

Monitoring blood sugar levels: To get the best possible glycemic control, periodically check your blood sugar levels to evaluate the effects of your food decisions and make any necessary modifications.

You may empower yourself to make educated dietary decisions that promote stable blood sugar levels, boost general health, and improve quality of life by becoming an expert on the GI & GL diabetic diet. You may effectively manage the complications of diabetes and make long-term progress toward improved health with commitment, knowledge, and useful techniques.

Grasping the Science-Backed Principles of the GI & GL Diet

The glycemic index (GI) and glycemic load (GL) diets are based on an abundance of scientific studies that show how various carbs affect blood sugar levels. Understanding the fundamentals of this diet enables people to make knowledgeable decisions about the foods they eat, which improves their capacity to control diseases like diabetes and enhances general health and well-being.

The foundation of the GI & GL diet is a knowledge of how the body breaks down and uses carbohydrates. The body uses carbs as its main energy source, but not all carbohydrates are made equally. Some cause abrupt rises in blood sugar levels because they are promptly converted to glucose and absorbed into the circulation. These foods have a high glycemic index (GI). Some, on the other hand, digest more slowly and release glucose into the circulation gradually and steadily. These foods have a low glycemic index (GI).

A food's glycemic load (GL) accounts for both the amount of carbs per serving and the food's glycemic index. This gives a more realistic impression of the impact a meal will have on blood sugar levels. People who prioritize meals with a low glycemic load may reduce blood glucose swings and sustain steady energy levels all day long.

The GI & GL diet's scientific basis emphasizes the value of selecting whole, minimally processed foods over highly refined and sweetened alternatives. In comparison to processed foods, whole grains, legumes, fruits, and vegetables are higher in fiber, vitamins, and minerals and have lower glycemic index and glycemic load values. Consuming these nutrient-dense meals may help people maintain optimum blood sugar management and advance their general health.

being aware of the GI & GL diet's tenets enables people to prepare pleasant, well-balanced meals that put long-term health results first. People may slow down the pace at which glucose enters the circulation and increase feelings of fullness and satisfaction by eating a diet high in fiber-rich vegetables, lean proteins, and healthy fats in addition to plenty of carbs. people may effectively control their blood sugar levels and improve their health by understanding the scientifically supported GI & GL diet guidelines.

People may minimize the risk of chronic illness, improve their general well-being, and promote stable energy levels by selecting nutrient-dense, low glycemic index, and glycemic-load meals.

Crafting Meals with Nutrient-Dense, Stable Blood Sugar Maintaining Foods

It's important to prioritize nutrient-dense products when creating meals that support stable blood sugar levels and enhance general health. You may prepare nutritious, well-balanced meals that enhance your health by choosing foods high in vital nutrients and keeping in mind how they affect blood glucose levels. Here's how you can begin:

Select Complex carbs: Try to steer clear of carbs with a high glycemic index (GI) and low fiber content. Whole grains like barley, quinoa, and brown rice are a few examples, along with starchy veggies like sweet potatoes and legumes like lentils and chickpeas. Because these complex carbs digest more slowly, blood sugar levels are stabilized and glucose is released into the circulation gradually.

Lean Proteins: Including lean protein sources in your meals may help control blood sugar levels and increase feelings of fullness. Select lean meats like turkey, chicken breast, and fish, as well as plant-based proteins like tempeh, tofu, and beans. foods high in protein may help reduce the speed at which carbs are absorbed and digested, reducing blood sugar rises that occur right after meals.

Add Healthy Fats: You may intensify the blood sugar-stabilizing benefits of your meals by including sources of healthy fats in them. Choose unsaturated fats, which are included in avocados, nuts, seeds, and olive oil, among other foods. These fats are a great supplement to your meals since they may increase insulin sensitivity and feel full.

Eat a lot of non-starchy vegetables: They are high in important vitamins, minerals, and antioxidants yet low in calories and carbs. Adding vibrant veggies to your meals—like broccoli, tomatoes, bell peppers, and leafy greens—will boost their nutritional content and volume without having a big effect on your blood sugar levels.

Maintain Portion Control: Although consuming meals high in nutrients is good for you, it's crucial to maintain portion control to prevent overindulging and blood sugar increases. Try to load your plate with three-quarters of complex carbs, one-quarter of lean protein, and half of non-starchy veggies. Pay attention to the signals your body gives you about when you are hungry and satisfied.

Make Whole, Unprocessed Foods a Priority: When organizing your meals, give special attention to minimally refined, whole, unprocessed foods that are devoid of artificial sweeteners and bad fats. Fruits, vegetables, whole grains, lean meats, and healthy fats are examples of foods that fit this description. These meals provide long-lasting energy without sharp spikes in blood sugar levels and are rich in vital nutrients.

You may promote optimum health and well-being while successfully controlling your diabetes by adhering to these recommendations and including nutrient-dense, stable blood sugar-maintaining foods in your meals.

To make tasty and fulfilling meals that feed your body and help you achieve your overall health objectives, try experimenting with various ingredients, tastes, and cooking techniques.

Embracing Healthier Alternatives to Manage Diabetes Effectively

Making deliberate dietary choices is frequently a necessary step on the path to optimum health for people with diabetes. Adopting better options may have a big impact on controlling blood sugar levels, lowering the chance of problems, and enhancing general health.

Emphasizing nutrient-dense, complete meals that are low in sugar and processed carbs is one of the fundamentals of good diabetic management. These more healthful options minimize the influence on blood glucose levels while still providing vital vitamins, minerals, and antioxidants. People with diabetes may have a balanced and fulfilling eating pattern that supports their health objectives by including a range of fruits, vegetables, whole grains, lean meats, and healthy fats in their diet. Choosing whole grains over processed grains is an easy but effective method to make better decisions when it comes to carbs. Compared to refined grains, whole grains like brown rice, quinoa, oats, and whole wheat are higher in fiber and minerals, which helps to maintain stable blood sugar levels and provide continuous energy throughout the day.

In a similar vein, selecting lean protein sources like lentils, fish, chicken, and tofu may boost muscle development and repair while assisting those with diabetes in controlling their blood sugar levels. These better options are also heart-healthy since they have less cholesterol and saturated fat than processed and red meat. Another smart way to properly manage diabetes is to include plenty of non-starchy veggies in meals and snacks. Leafy greens, broccoli, cauliflower, and peppers are examples of vegetables that are low in calories and carbs yet high in fiber, vitamins, and minerals. They provide color, taste, and nutritional content to any dish and may be eaten raw or prepared in a multitude of delectable ways.

Good fats, like those in nuts, seeds, avocados, and olive oil, are also a crucial component of a diet that is diabetes-friendly. These more healthful options include vital fatty acids that enhance insulin sensitivity, lower inflammation, and promote brain function. By adding these fats to meals and snacks, people may maintain stable blood sugar levels and feel full and content.

Effective diabetes management includes eating a better diet, drinking enough of water, and paying attention to portion sizes. Being aware of portion sizes helps avoid overeating and maintains blood sugar levels while drinking plenty of water throughout the day promotes general health and hydration.

Adopting healthier substitutes is essential to properly controlling diabetes.

People with diabetes may take charge of their health and lead happy, active lives by making nutrient-dense, whole-food choices and paying attention to portion sizes.

Diabetes management may become a journey towards improved health and well-being, rather than simply a medical need, with commitment, knowledge, and support.

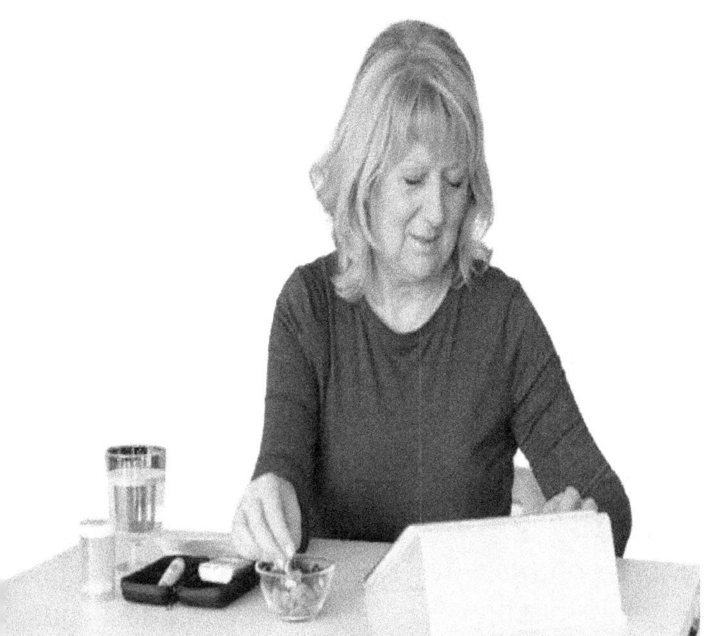

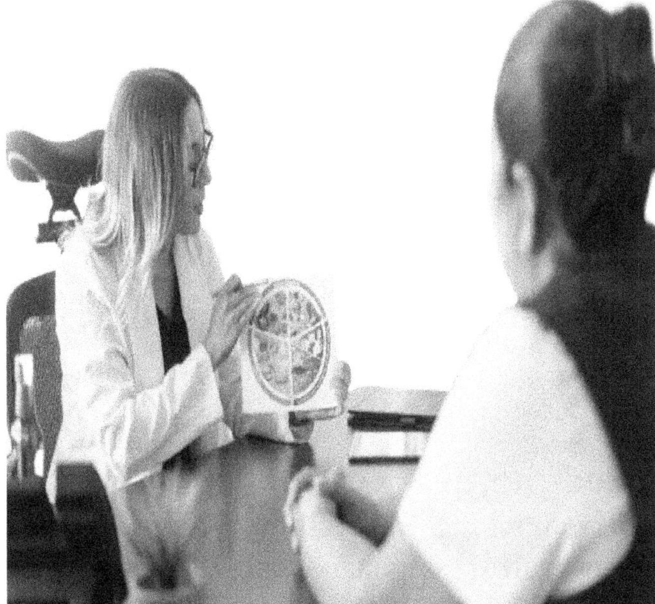

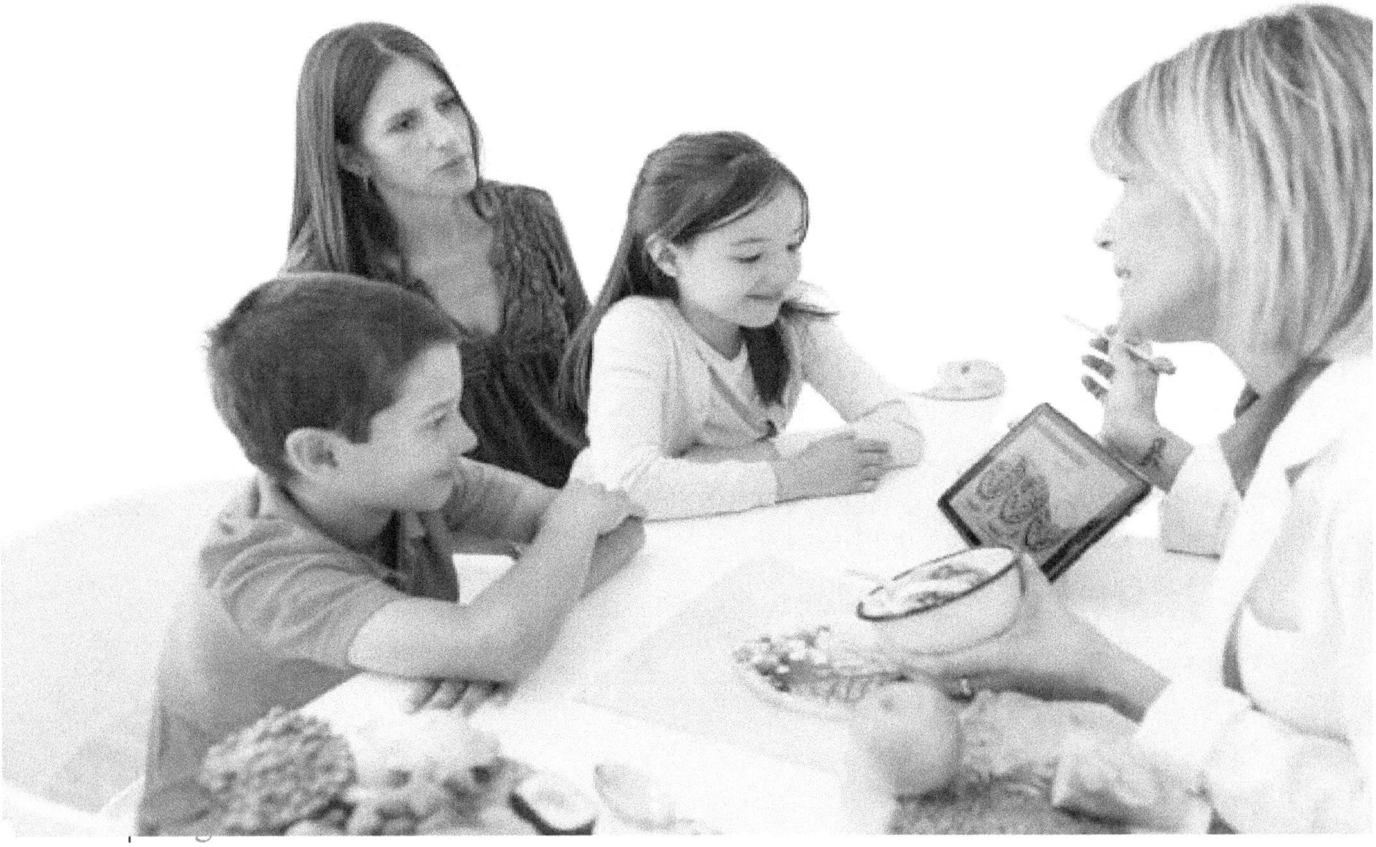

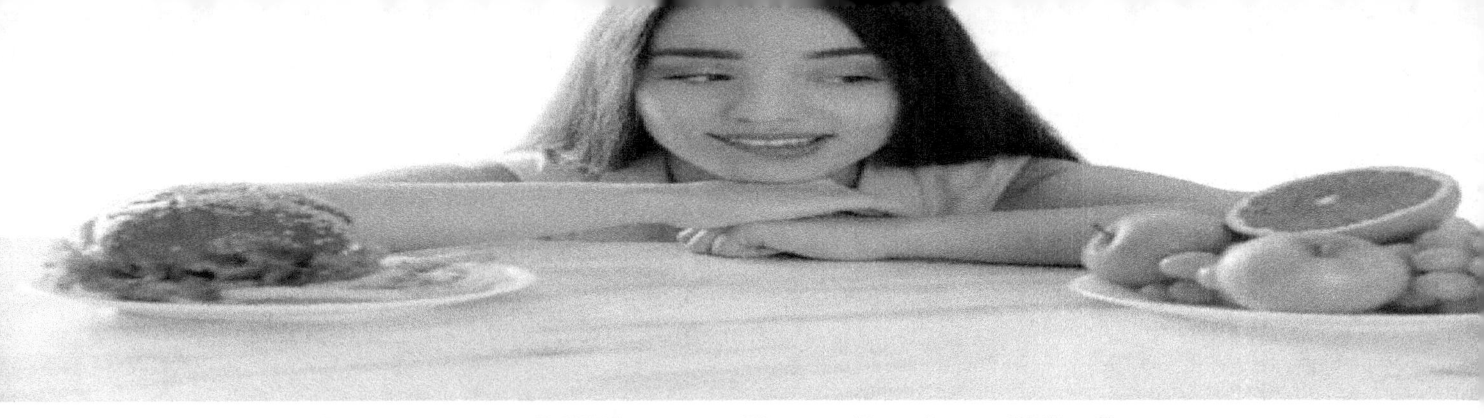

Best and Worst Foods for Diabetes

Making dietary decisions and navigating the shopping aisles may be difficult, particularly for those who are managing their diabetes. Maintaining stable blood sugar levels and enhancing general health need an understanding of which meals are healthy and which ones are best avoided.

To assist you in making wise dietary choices, we'll go over some of the greatest and worst foods for diabetes in this section.

Top Diabetes-Friendly Foods

Non-Starchy Vegetables: High in fiber, vitamins, and minerals, but low in calories and carbs, vegetables like leafy greens, broccoli, cauliflower, peppers, and cucumbers are a good choice. They aid in filling you full without giving you noticeable blood sugar rises.

Whole Grains: Including whole grains in your diet, such as quinoa, brown rice, barley, and oats, releases glucose into your circulation more gradually due to their slower digestion.

Lean Proteins: Without adding an excessive amount of cholesterol or saturated fat, lean protein sources including fish, chicken, tofu, and lentils may help control blood sugar levels and encourage fullness.

Healthy Fats: Since heart disease is often more common in people with diabetes, foods high in healthy fats, such as avocados, nuts, seeds, and olive oil, may enhance insulin sensitivity and lower the risk of cardiovascular disease.

Low-Glycemic Fruits: When eaten in moderation, fruits including berries, apples, cherries, citrus fruits, and walnuts are better for people with diabetes since they have more fiber and less sugar.

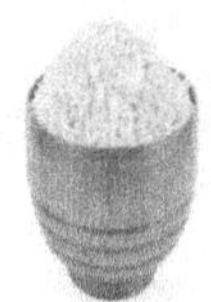
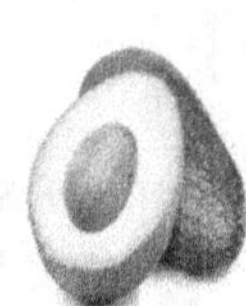
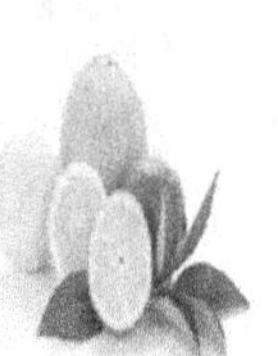
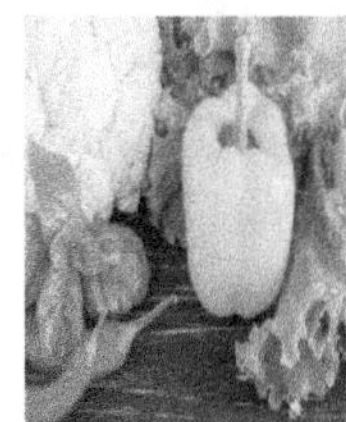

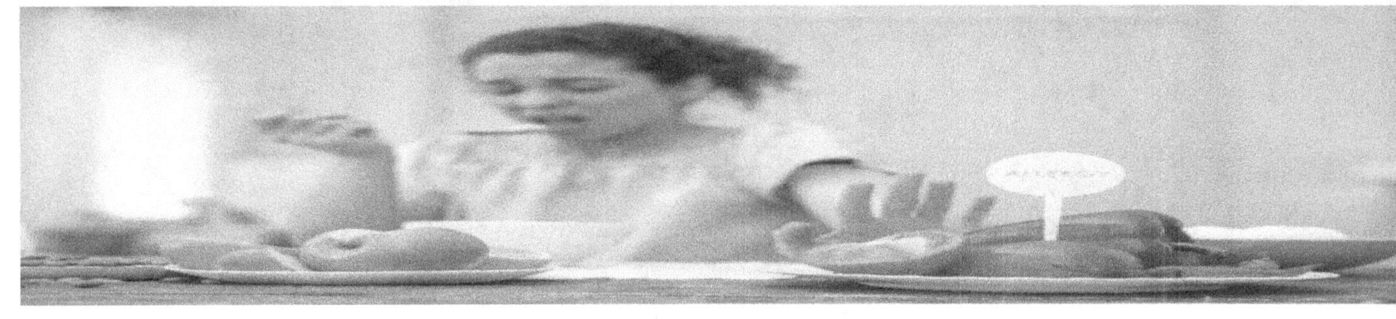

Sugary beverages: Sugary beverages, such as carbonated tea, fruit juices, energy drinks, and soda, are bad for managing diabetes since they may quickly raise blood sugar levels and lead to weight gain.

Processed Foods: It is best to minimize or stay away from processed foods that are heavy in added sugars, refined carbs, and harmful fats. White bread, pastries, sugary cereals, and packaged snacks are a few examples.

Fried Foods: Fried foods, such as doughnuts, fried chicken, and French fries, are heavy in calories and bad fats, which increases the risk of cardiovascular problems and insulin resistance in diabetics.

Full-Fat Dairy: Although dairy products are a good addition to a balanced diet, full-fat types, such as cheese, ice cream, and whole milk, contain saturated fats that may increase cholesterol and cause insulin resistance.

Rich-salt Foods: Consuming foods rich in salt, such as canned soups, processed meats, and fast food, may boost blood pressure and heart disease risk, which is already higher in diabetics.

Individuals may enhance their general health and well-being, lower the risk of problems, and better control their blood sugar levels by being aware of the best and worst diets for diabetes and intentionally prioritizing nutrient-rich selections.

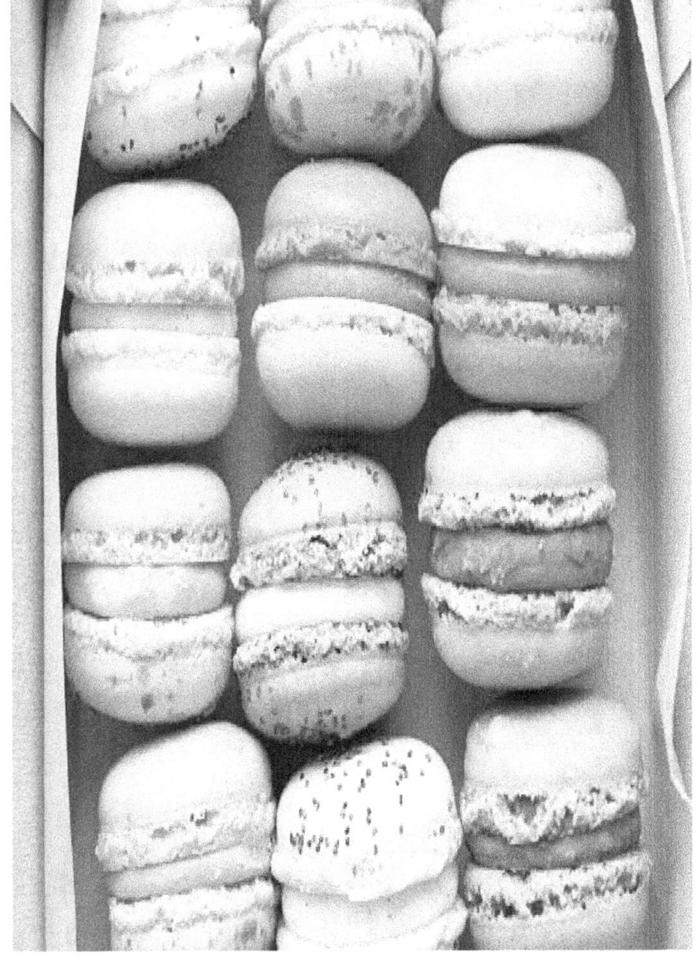

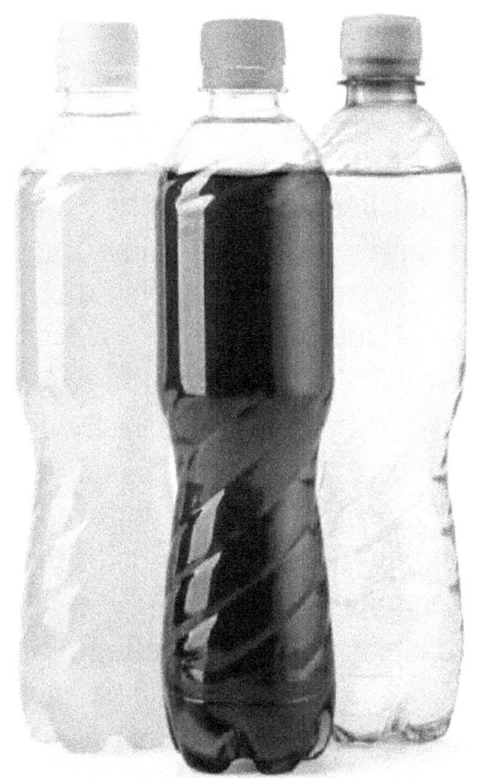

It's important to know which foods are suitable for a diabetic diet and which ones are not, according to a health and wellness expert who is passionate about providing people with the information they need to live healthy lives. The identification of these foods and how to choose wisely to promote optimum health and well-being will be covered in this part.

Foods that are low-glycemic and high in nutrients without producing large rises in blood sugar are considered diabetes-friendly meals. These consist of:

Non-starchy veggies: You may receive important vitamins, minerals, and fiber from foods like peppers, cucumbers, and tomatoes, as well as cruciferous vegetables and other non-starchy vegetables, without having a major impact on blood sugar levels.

Whole grains: Because they digest more slowly and have a greater fiber content than refined grains, whole grains like quinoa, brown rice, oats, and barley help control blood sugar levels.

Lean protein: Lean protein foods, such as fish, chicken, tofu, lentils, and eggs, may support muscle function and repair while also helping to balance blood sugar levels and encourage satiety.

Healthy fats: Incorporating sources of healthy fats such as avocados, nuts, seeds, and olive oil can help slow down the absorption of carbohydrates and promote feelings of fullness, making them valuable additions to a diabetes-friendly diet.

Contrarily, meals that are considered non-compliant may result in sharp rises in blood sugar levels, as well as an increased risk of insulin resistance and other diabetes-related problems. These consist of:

Refined carbohydrates: Foods made with white flour, sugar, and other refined carbohydrates, such as white bread, pastries, sugary cereals, and sweetened beverages, should be limited or avoided as they can lead to sharp increases in blood sugar levels.

Sugary snacks and desserts: Processed snacks, candies, cookies, cakes, and other sugary treats are high in refined sugars and provide little to no nutritional value, making them detrimental to blood sugar control and overall health.

Meals rich in fat and processed: Products like fried meals, processed meats, and premade snacks should be consumed in moderation since they raise the risk of heart disease and insulin resistance.

By becoming familiar with these guidelines and learning to identify diabetes-friendly and non-compliant foods, you can make empowered choices that support your health and well-being. It is important to keep in mind that little adjustments may have a big impact on blood sugar regulation and general well-being.

Understanding the Impact of Food Choices on Glucose Levels

The key to managing diabetes is controlling blood glucose levels, and one of the biggest variables affecting blood sugar levels is what we eat. We will dig into the complex link between dietary choices and blood glucose levels in this extensive educational discourse, examining how certain nutrients and dietary patterns impact glycemic management. People may enhance their health and well-being by making educated food selections by having a complete awareness of these principles.

The Function of Carbohydrates: The main macronutrient influencing blood glucose levels is carbohydrates, which may be found in a variety of meals including grains, fruits, vegetables, dairy products, and sweets. Carbohydrates are converted in the body into glucose, which enters the circulation and elevates blood sugar. The kind and quantity of carbs taken in are important factors in figuring out how much of an increase this is.

Glycemic Index and Glycemic Load: The glycemic index (GI) and glycemic load (GL) are two essential ideas in comprehending how carbohydrates affect blood glucose levels. The glycemic load accounts for both the amount and quality of carbohydrates in a serving of food, while the glycemic index gauges how rapidly a carbohydrate-containing item elevates blood sugar levels in comparison to a reference food. Blood sugar levels rise more gradually with foods having a low GI or GL than they do with foods with a high GI or GL.

Fiber and Blood Sugar Regulation: The body is unable to absorb fiber, a kind of carbohydrate that is included in plant-based diets. Rather, it travels through the digestive tract mostly undisturbed, which lessens the effect on blood sugar levels and slows down the absorption of glucose. Eating a diet high in fruits, vegetables, whole grains, legumes, and nuts may help lower blood sugar levels and enhance glycemic management in general.

Protein and Fat: Although carbs affect blood glucose levels the most, protein and fat also contribute to glycemic management. After meals, blood sugar levels increase more gradually because protein and fat slow down the digestion and absorption of carbs. Including foods like chicken, fish, tofu, nuts, seeds, and avocado that are high in lean protein and healthy fats will help stabilize blood sugar levels and increase feelings of fullness.

Meal Timing and Composition: Blood glucose levels are also influenced by the timing and makeup of meals. Regularly consuming well-balanced meals and snacks spread out throughout the day may aid in preventing blood sugar swings. Carbohydrates may also be better paired with protein, fat, and fiber to improve glycemic control by lowering post-meal spikes and slowing down glucose absorption.

successful diabetes treatment requires an understanding of how dietary decisions affect blood glucose levels. Through the use of glycemic index, glycemic load, fiber consumption, and meal composition as

Individual Variability: It's important to understand that a person's reaction to food may differ significantly depending on several variables, including insulin sensitivity, medication usage, degree of physical activity, and general health. A person may not have the same results from something that works well for them. As a result, people with diabetes must constantly check their blood glucose levels, try new foods and meal schedules, and collaborate closely with medical specialists to create individualized diet programs.

guiding principles in one's diet, people may enhance blood sugar regulation, lower their risk of problems, and enhance their general health and well-being. To achieve ideal glycemic control and have a healthy life with diabetes, education, experimentation, and cooperation with healthcare professionals are essential.

Creating Awareness about Beneficial and Harmful Foods in a Diabetic Diet

Knowing how various meals affect blood sugar levels is one of the most important skills in managing the complicated world of diabetes. Making educated food choices may make the difference between hazardous swings in blood sugar levels and consistent management, which can lead to major health issues for those with diabetes. Thus, educating people about the good and bad foods to include in a diabetic diet is crucial to giving them the confidence to take charge of their health and well-being.

Good Foods:

Non-Starchy veggies: For those with diabetes, non-starchy veggies including bell peppers, cucumbers, broccoli, cauliflower, and leafy greens are great options. They are excellent for boosting satiety and regulating blood sugar levels since they are low in calories and carbs and abundant in fiber, vitamins, and minerals.

Whole Grains: Packed with fiber and complex carbs, whole grains like quinoa, brown rice, oats, and barley digest more slowly than refined grains. This slow digestion gives you steady energy throughout the day and helps avoid sharp increases in blood sugar.

Lean Proteins: An essential part of a diabetic diet includes lean protein sources, which include skinless chicken, fish, tofu, beans, and lentils. Protein slows down the absorption of carbs and increases feelings of fullness, both of which may assist with blood sugar regulation and weight control.

Good Fats: Good fats, which are included in foods like avocados, nuts, seeds, and olive oil, may aid diabetics with insulin sensitivity and lower their chance of developing cardiovascular disease. These fats may also improve taste and enjoyment without significantly raising blood sugar levels when added to meals and snacks.

Unhealthy Foods:

Refined carbs: A diabetic diet should restrict or completely avoid foods prepared with refined carbs, such as white bread, white rice, sugary cereals, pastries, and sugary drinks. These meals have a high rate of digestion and may raise blood sugar levels rapidly, resulting in spikes and crashes.

Sugary Snacks and Desserts: In addition to being low in nutrients, foods heavy in added sugars, such as candy, cookies, cakes, and sweetened drinks, also lead to unhealthful weight gain and poor blood sugar regulation. Diabetes sufferers should choose healthier options or indulge in these delicacies sparingly.

Fried and processed foods: Fried foods, fast food, frozen dinners, and packaged snacks are examples of processed foods that are rich in salt, bad fats, and added sugars that may be detrimental to blood sugar regulation and general health. Particularly fried meals should be restricted in a diabetic diet since they are heavy in calories and harmful fats.

Rich-Sodium Foods: Consuming foods rich in sodium, such as canned soups, processed meats, and salty snacks, may raise blood pressure and put diabetics at risk for cardiovascular problems. Reducing salt consumption and promoting heart health may be achieved by selecting low-sodium substitutes and enhancing meals with herbs and spices.

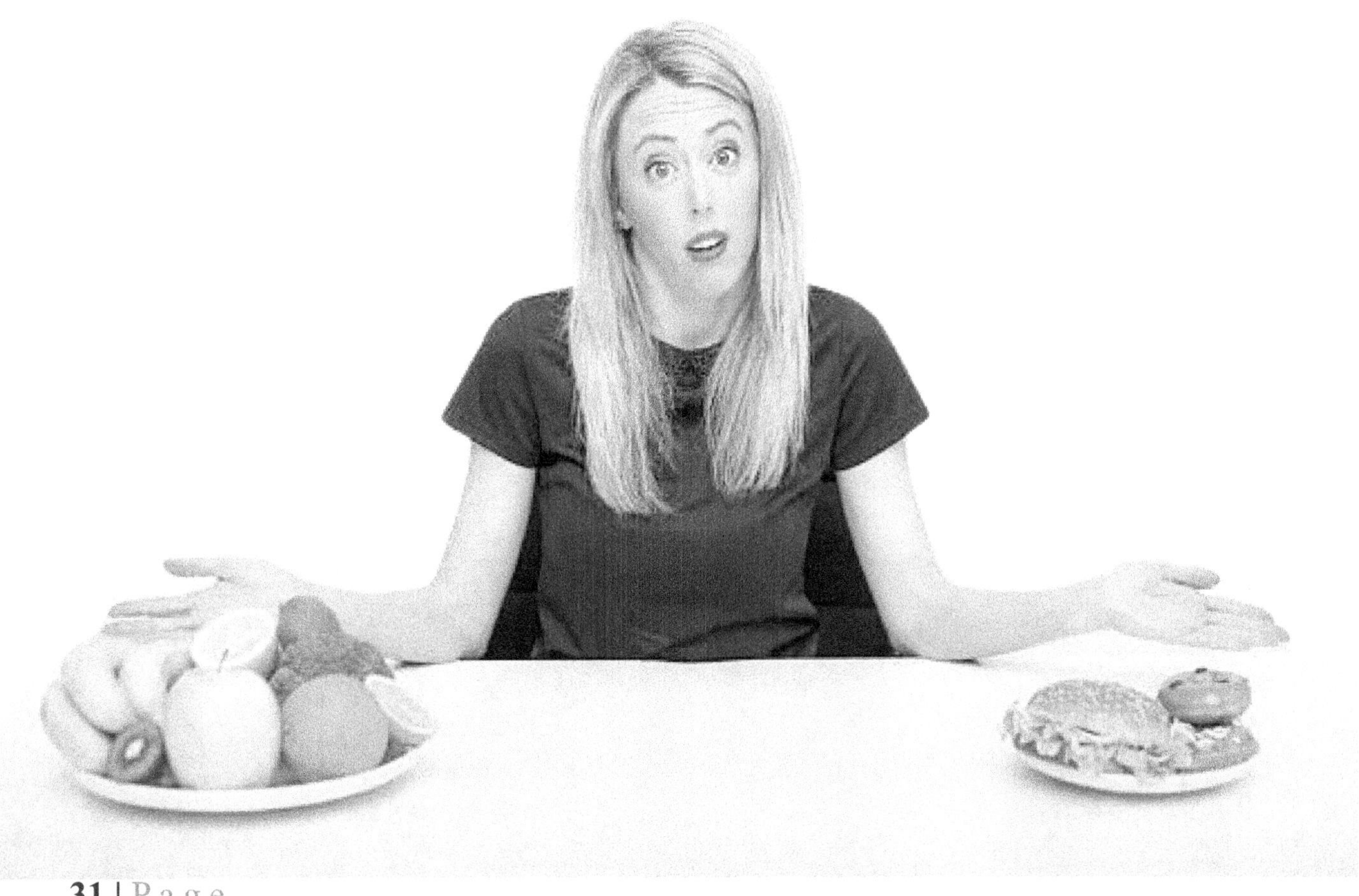

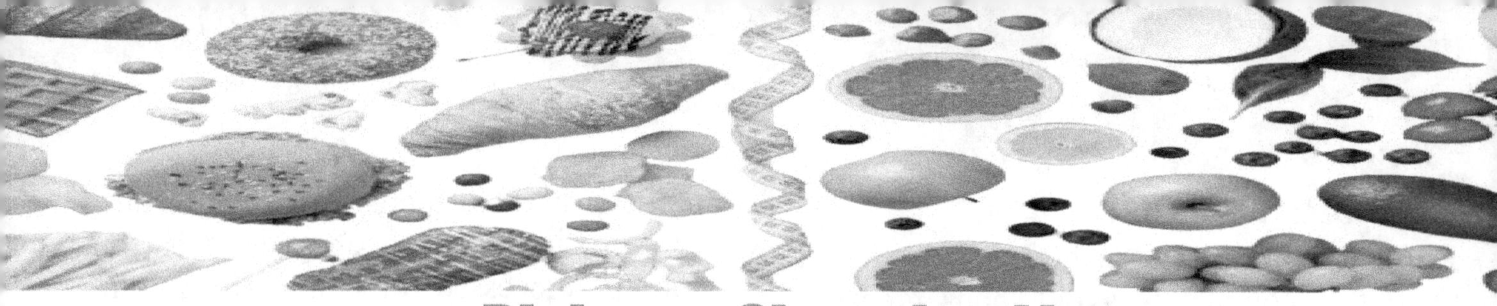

Diabetes Shopping List

Produce:
1. Leafy greens (spinach, kale, arugula)
2. Cruciferous vegetables (broccoli, cauliflower, Brussels sprouts)
3. Bell peppers (red, green, yellow)
4. Cucumbers
5. Tomatoes
6. Carrots
7. Celery
8. Zucchini
9. Onions
10. Garlic

Fruits:
1. Berries (strawberries, blueberries, raspberries)
2. Apples
3. Pears
4. Oranges
5. Grapefruit
6. Kiwi
7. Cherries
8. Peaches
9. Plums
10. Avocado

Grains and Legumes:
1. Quinoa
2. Brown rice
3. Whole wheat pasta
4. Oats
5. Lentils
6. Chickpeas
7. Black beans
6. Pumpkin seeds
8. Kidney beans
9. Farro
10. Barley

Proteins:
1. Skinless chicken breast
2. Turkey breast
3. Salmon
4. Tuna
5. Tofu
6. Eggs
7. Greek yogurt (unsweetened)
8. Cottage cheese (low-fat)
9. Lean cuts of beef or pork
10. Tempeh

Dairy and Dairy Alternatives:
1. Low-fat milk
2. Unsweetened almond milk
3. Low-fat cheese
4. Plain yogurt (low-fat)
5. Kefir
6. Ricotta cheese (part-skim)
7. Soy milk (unsweetened)
8. Greek yogurt (plain, unsweetened)
9. Cottage cheese (low-fat)
10. Non-dairy yogurt alternatives (unsweetened)

Nuts and Seeds:
1. Almonds
2. Walnuts
3. Cashews
4. Chia seeds
5. Flaxseeds
6. Dark chocolate (at least 70% cocoa)

7. Sunflower seeds
8. Pistachios
9. Hemp seeds
10. Sesame seeds

Miscellaneous:

1. Olive oil
2. Avocado oil
3. Vinegar (balsamic, apple cider, red wine)
4. Herbs and spices (basil, oregano, cinnamon, turmeric)
5. Low-sodium broth (vegetable, chicken)

7. Unsweetened cocoa powder
8. Canned tomatoes (no added sugar)
9. Sugar-free condiments (mustard, salsa, hot sauce)
10. Whole grain bread or wraps

Remember to prioritize whole, unprocessed foods and check food labels for added sugars and unhealthy fats. Planning your meals and snacks around these nutritious ingredients will help support stable blood sugar levels and overall health in individuals with diabetes.

Navigating Grocery Aisles with Confidence

Grocery shopping may provide chances for people with diabetes to make health-promoting decisions, as well as some specific hurdles. Diabetes patients may choose foods that support stable blood sugar levels and enhance general well-being by carefully planning ahead and gaining a little knowledge to make grocery shopping an empowering experience.

Here are some helpful hints to help diabetics confidently traverse supermarket aisles:

Plan Ahead: Invest some time in organizing your weekly menu before you go to the supermarket. List the things you must eat, emphasizing nutrient-dense foods like fruits, vegetables, whole grains, lean meats, and healthy fats. You can remain organized and prevent impulsive purchases of less healthy goods by making a plan in advance.

Examine labels: Pay close attention to the nutrition labels when you shop for packaged items. Observe the amount of carbohydrates in total as well as the size and quantity of servings in each container. Choose meals that minimally processed meals that are as near to

are rich in fiber and low in added sugars since they are often better options for controlling blood sugar levels.

Select Fresh Produce: The produce department is a diabetic's greatest ally. For maximum nutritious advantages, use a range of colors and textures when packing on the fresh fruits and veggies. Fruit juices and canned fruits coated in syrup should be avoided in favor of whole fruits, since the latter may have less fiber and more sugar.

Choose Whole Grains: Go for whole grain products whenever you can when buying cereals and grains. Aim for "whole grain" or "whole wheat" items; stay away from processed grains, such as those found in sweet cereals and white bread and rice. Because whole grains are high in minerals and fiber, they may help control blood sugar levels and strengthen heart health.

Eat Less Processed Foods: Processed and packaged foods should be avoided since they often include high levels of added sugars, salt, and harmful fats. Rather, prioritize whole,

Be Flexible: It's OK to sometimes indulge

their original condition as feasible. Products like fresh meats, poultry, fish, eggs, and dairy are included in this.

Practice Portion Control: When choosing meals, particularly those heavy in carbohydrates like bread, pasta, and rice, be mindful of portion proportions. To assist regulate portion sizes at home, use measuring cups and spoons to measure out food and think about using smaller plates and bowls.

in moderation even though it's crucial to make healthy decisions the majority of the time. Give yourself permission to indulge in your favorite goodies sometimes, but watch the quantity that you consume and how they affect your blood sugar levels.

Selecting the Right Foods for Diabetes-Friendly Options

For people with diabetes, making the appropriate dietary choices is essential since nutrition is a major factor in both blood sugar regulation and general health. Choosing diabetes-friendly foods may assist people in controlling their blood sugar levels, maintaining a healthy weight, and lowering their chance of developing complications from the disease. Here are some helpful tips for choosing the best meals for diabetic-friendly options:

Stress Whole, Unprocessed meals: Packed with fiber and other minerals, whole, unprocessed meals may help control blood sugar levels and increase fullness. Make an effort to increase your intake of entire grains, fruits, vegetables, lean meats, and healthy fats. These nutrient-dense meals provide a consistent energy boost without sharp jumps in blood sugar levels.

Observe Carbohydrate Quantity and Quality: Since carbs have the biggest effect on blood sugar levels, it's critical to pay attention to the quantity and quality of carbohydrates you eat. Choose complex carbs with a lower glycemic index, such as those found in whole grains, legumes, and non-starchy vegetables. These foods also digest more slowly. Furthermore, portion management is essential since even healthful carbs may impact blood sugar levels if ingested in excess.

Select Lean Protein Sources: Because it encourages feelings of fullness and helps control blood sugar levels, protein is a crucial food for people with diabetes. To reduce saturated fat consumption and promote general heart health, choose lean protein sources such skinless chicken, fish, tofu, beans, and lentils. Including protein with every meal may help control blood sugar levels and avoid insulin production spikes.

Include Good Fats: Good fats are essential to a diabetes-friendly diet since they increase heart health and insulin sensitivity. Olive oil, avocados, almonds, seeds, and fatty fish like trout and salmon are good sources of both monounsaturated and polyunsaturated fats. These fats may improve general metabolic performance, decrease cholesterol, and lessen inflammation.

You may make proactive moves toward improved blood sugar management and

Analyze Food Labels and Ingredients Lists: It's critical to thoroughly examine food labels and ingredient lists while choosing packaged and processed foods. Seek products with whole food components and little processing, and steer clear of those high in salt, bad fats, and added sweets. Make sure that the foods you choose fit your dietary requirements and objectives by keeping an eye on serving sizes and carbohydrate levels.

Use Mindful Eating and Portion Control: Reducing portion size is essential for controlling blood sugar levels and avoiding overindulgence. At each meal, try to fill half of your plate with non-starchy veggies by using measuring cups, spoons, and food scales to divide out quantities of carbs, proteins, and fats. Eat mindfully by observing your body's signals of hunger and fullness, taking your time, and enjoying every mouthful.

general health by choosing diabetes-friendly foods and implementing these educational techniques into your meal plans. Recall that little, long-lasting adjustments build up over time, and adopting wise dietary choices may have big long-term effects on your health.

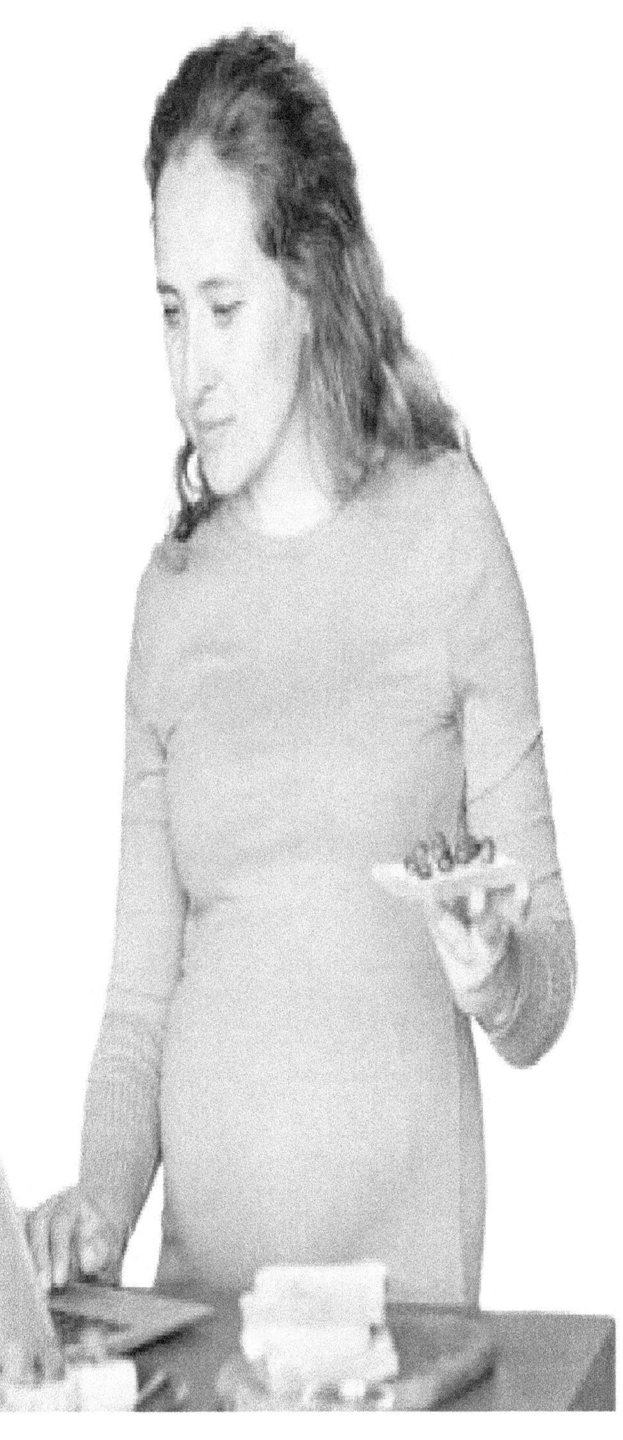

Grocery shopping list

<table>
<tr><td>

☐ ______________________
☐ ______________________
☐ ______________________
☐ ______________________
☐ ______________________
☐ ______________________
☐ ______________________
☐ ______________________
☐ ______________________
☐ ______________________
☐ ______________________
☐ ______________________
☐ ______________________
☐ ______________________
☐ ______________________
☐ ______________________
☐ ______________________
☐ ______________________
☐ ______________________
☐ ______________________
☐ ______________________
☐ ______________________
☐ ______________________
☐ ______________________
☐ ______________________
☐ ______________________
☐ ______________________
☐ ______________________
☐ ______________________

</td><td>

Fruits and Vegetable

☐ ______________________
☐ ______________________
☐ ______________________
☐ ______________________
☐ ______________________
☐ ______________________
☐ ______________________
☐ ______________________
☐ ______________________

Meat / Poultry / Fish

☐ ______________________
☐ ______________________
☐ ______________________
☐ ______________________
☐ ______________________
☐ ______________________
☐ ______________________
☐ ______________________

Grains

☐ ______________________
☐ ______________________
☐ ______________________
☐ ______________________
☐ ______________________
☐ ______________________
☐ ______________________
☐ ______________________

</td></tr>
</table>

Grocery shopping list

Making wise selections for a better lifestyle is a complex process that entails prioritizing health-promoting actions and realizing how our everyday choices affect our general well-being. Every decision we make, whether it's about eating healthily, getting regular exercise, controlling our stress levels, or building a network of supporting people, may either improve or worsen our quality of life.

Eating a balanced, nutrient-rich diet is one of the fundamentals of making decisions that will help you live a better life. This means choosing a range of entire foods that are high in vital elements including antioxidants, fiber, vitamins, and minerals. Focusing on nutrient-dense foods such as fruits, vegetables, whole grains, lean proteins, and healthy fats, people may promote optimum physiological performance and feed their bodies.

knowing how various foods affect our health outcomes is essential for making educated dietary decisions, especially for those who are managing chronic diseases like diabetes, heart disease, or obesity. Through knowledge of terms like glycemic load (GL), glycemic index (GI), and portion management, people may adjust how they eat to better regulate blood sugar, support heart health, and reach or maintain a healthy weight.

Making educated decisions for a better lifestyle includes not just diet but also physical exercise, stress reduction, good sleep hygiene, and social support. For example, regular exercise not only strengthens the body and improves cardiovascular health, but it also elevates mood, lowers stress levels, and encourages higher-quality sleep.

In a similar vein, reducing stress via methods like deep breathing exercises, mindfulness meditation, or time spent in nature may have a significant positive impact on mental and physical health. A proper sleep schedule and getting enough sleep are also vital for general health as sleep is necessary for immunological response, mental clarity, and emotional control.

cultivating positive social relationships and maintaining a robust support system may enhance resistance to life's obstacles and facilitate a feeling of acceptance and contentment.

Taking a proactive and comprehensive approach to health and well-being is ultimately what it means to make educated decisions for a healthy lifestyle. We can empower ourselves to live bright, meaningful lives and succeed in all areas of our lives by learning about the variables that affect our health and putting methods into place to promote optimum living.

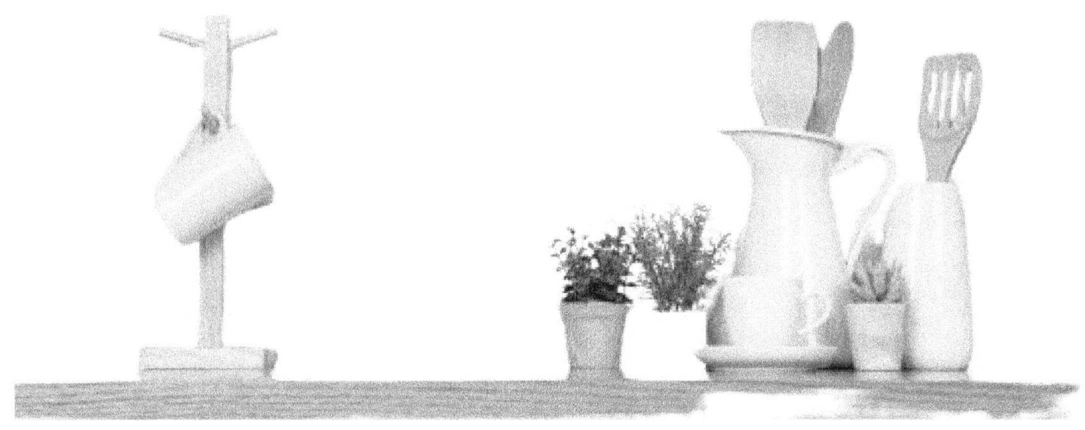

Detailed Meal Planning Guidelines

|--------------------
| **Step 1:** Assess
| Current Diet
| and Preferences
|--------------------
| **Step 3: Plan**
| Balanced Meals
|--------------------
| - Include a variety
| of food groups
| - Aim for nutrient
| density
| - Consider portion
| sizes
|--------------------
| **Step 5: Make a**
|
| **Shopping List**
|--------------------
| - Compile a list of
| necessary ingredients
| - Check pantry and
| refrigerator for
| staples

|-----------------------------------|
| **Step 2: Set Goals** |
| - Determine nutritional goals |
| - Identify dietary restrictions |
-|-----------------------------------|
| **Step 4: Create Meal** |
| Templates |
-|------------------------------------|
| - Designate meals for each |
| day of the week |
| - Incorporate balance of |
| macronutrients |
| - Include options for |
| customization |
| |-------------------------------------|
| **Step 6: Prepare Ingredients**
|
| **and Precook** |
|-------------------------------------|
| - Wash, chop, and portion |
| ingredients |
| - Precook staples such as |
| grains, proteins, and veggies |
| - Store in meal prep containers |

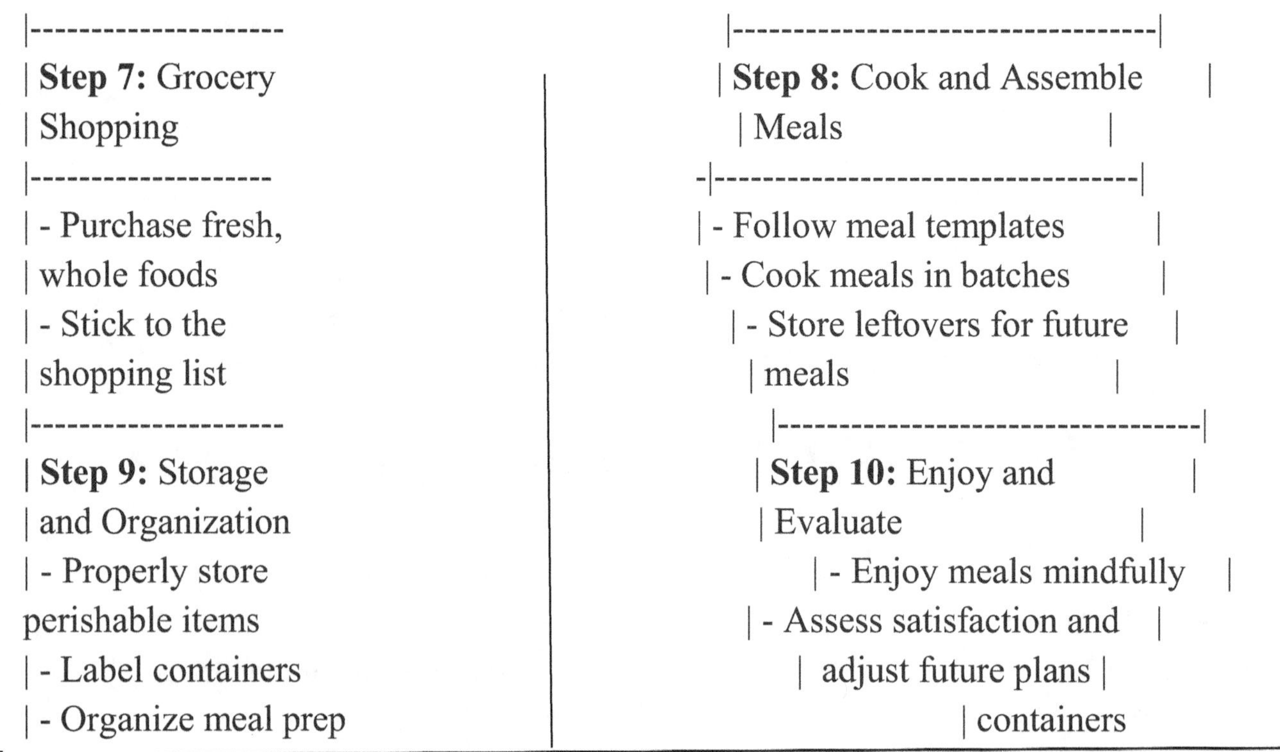

Guidelines for Each Major Food Group for Simplified Meal Preparation

Produce:

When preparing meals, try to include a range of non-starchy vegetables, such as tomatoes, bell peppers, broccoli, cauliflower, and leafy greens.

To guarantee that you are getting enough fiber and nutrients without having a major effect on your blood sugar levels, put half of your plate on veggies.

Try varied cooking techniques, such as sautéing, roasting, or steaming, to bring out the taste without using a lot of oil or salt.

When using starchy vegetables in your meal, choose smaller servings and steer clear of potatoes, peas, and corn.

Proteins:

Pick lean protein sources including fish, tofu, tempeh, skinless chicken, lentils, and low-fat dairy.

cards, but be aware of portion sizes.

Steer clear of high-fat foods and processed meats since they may increase cardiovascular risk factors.

Complete Grains:

To increase fiber content and decrease the pace at which carbs are absorbed and digested, choose whole grains over processed grains.

Select whole-grain bread, brown rice, quinoa, barley, oats, and whole-wheat pasta.

Aim for ½ to 1 cup of cooked whole grains every meal, monitoring portion amounts based on personal carbohydrate tolerance.

Try blending various grains into salads, soups, stir-fries, and grain bowls to add some variation to your meals.

Fruits:

Fresh, whole fruits are preferable since they

Include protein with every meal to help with blood sugar stabilization and fullness.

Aim for 3–4 ounces of cooked protein every meal, or approximately the size of a deck of pears, and citrus fruits.

To avoid blood sugar spikes, keep portion amounts in check and try to incorporate fruit in a balanced meal or snack.

To lessen the influence of fruits on blood sugar levels, think about combining them with protein or healthy fats.

Good Fats:

Include foods high in avocados, almonds, seeds, olive oil, and fatty fish like trout or salmon in your diet as sources of healthful fats.

When using fats and oils in cooking, use moderation and strive for small quantities to boost taste and satisfaction without adding extra calories.

have more fiber and less concentrated sugar than fruit juices or dried fruits.

Pay attention to fruits with a lower glycemic index, such as melons, berries, apples,

Because lipids are high in calories and may cause weight gain if ingested in excess, it is important to watch portion proportions.

As they raise the risk of heart disease, restrict and stay away from trans fats and saturated fats, which are present in processed meals, fried foods, and high-fat dairy products.

Following these recommendations will help you maintain optimum blood sugar management and general health as a diabetic while making meal preparation easier. Nutrient-dense foods from each major food category should be included in your meals.

Enhancing Meal Planning for Optimal Diabetes Management

The ability to proactively regulate one's blood sugar levels and general health is provided by meal planning, which is a fundamental component of successful diabetes treatment. People with diabetes may maximize their nutritional intake and lower their chance of problems by carefully choosing and preparing meals that support stable glucose levels. Here are a few essential tactics to improve meal planning for the best possible control of diabetes:

Prioritize Balanced Nutrition: All food categories should be included in a well-rounded meal plan, with an emphasis on nutrient-dense foods such as fruits, vegetables, whole grains, lean meats, and which are rich in vitamins, minerals, and antioxidants.

Measure and Control Carbohydrate Consumption: Meal planning must include monitoring and controlling carbohydrate consumption since carbohydrates have the most effect on blood sugar levels. To make sure that your daily intake of carbohydrates is steady and well-balanced, think about using carb counting or portion management techniques. Select carbs that have a low glycemic load (GL) and GI to reduce blood sugar rises.

Incorporate Lean Proteins: Protein helps to maintain blood sugar levels and to induce sensations of fullness and satiety. To help

healthy fats. Choose whole grains over processed carbs to encourage satiety and stable blood sugar levels. Aim to include a diverse variety of fruits and vegetables,

Insist on Healthy Fats: For people with diabetes, healthy fats—like those in nuts, seeds, avocados, and olive oil—can help increase insulin sensitivity and lower their risk of heart disease. Add flavor and improve satiety to meals and snacks by using tiny amounts of healthy fats that won't drastically affect blood sugar levels.

Eat in Moderation: Portion management is essential for controlling blood sugar levels and calorie consumption, particularly for diabetics who may be at risk of weight gain or consequences from obesity. To portion out the right amounts of each food category and prevent overindulging, use measuring cups, food scales, or visual clues.

Plan and Be Flexible: Making better food choices and avoiding impulsive or unhealthy food choices may be achieved by people with diabetes who plan their meals. To expedite the process and lessen the temptation to stray from dietary objectives, set aside sometime each week to establish a meal plan, compile a shopping list, and prepare meals and snacks in advance. Being adaptive and flexible is also crucial, however, as unforeseen events might force alterations to the meal plan.

regulate blood sugar levels and avoid overindulging, include lean protein sources like fish, chicken, tofu, lentils, and low-fat dairy products in meals and snacks.

Monitor Blood Sugar Levels: To determine if meal planning tactics are helpful and to make the required changes, regular blood sugar monitoring is needed. For individualized advice and assistance, speak with a healthcare professional or qualified dietitian. Record your blood sugar levels before and after meals to see patterns and changes over time.

People with diabetes may take proactive measures towards better blood sugar control, general health, and quality of life by implementing these ideas into their meal planning routine. As you plan and prepare meals for diabetes control, keep in mind that moderation, balance, and consistency are important guidelines.

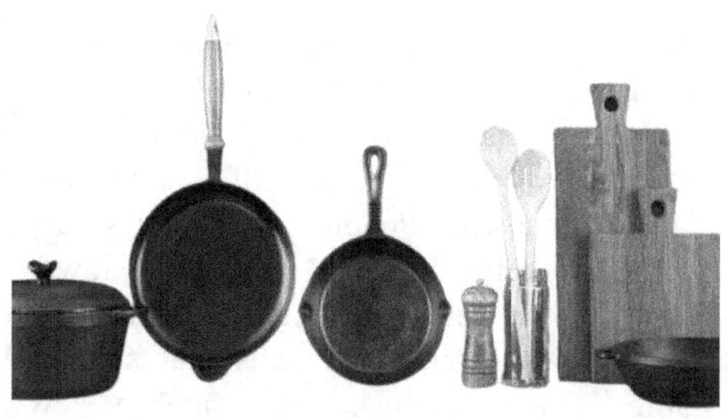

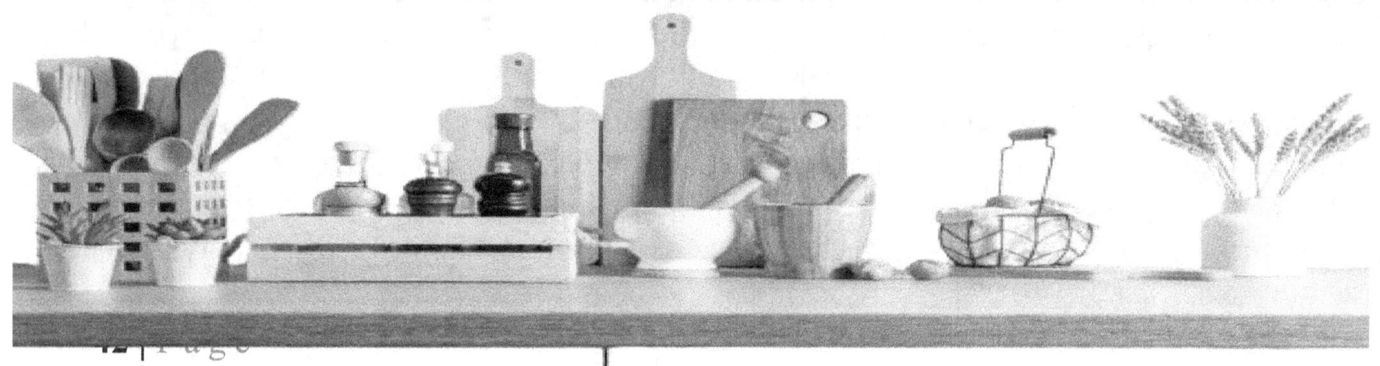

Tailored Recommendations

Apples
Apricots
Artichokes
Asparagus
Avocado
Bamboo shoots
Barley
Beans (black, kidney, pinto)
Beet greens
Bell peppers (green, red, yellow)
Berries (strawberries, blueberries, raspberries)
Bok choy
Broccoli
Brussels sprouts
Cabbage (green, red, Napa)
Carrots
Cauliflower
Celery
Cherries
Chickpeas
Collard greens
Cucumber
Eggplant
Endive
Fennel
Flaxseeds
Garlic
Grapefruit
Grapes
Green beans
Kale
Kiwi
Leeks
Lentils

Lettuce (all varieties)
Lima beans
Mushrooms (all varieties)
Mustard greens
Nectarines
Okra
Onions (all varieties)
Oranges
Papaya
Parsnips
Peaches
Peas (all varieties)
Pears
Pineapple
Plums
Pumpkin
Radishes
Raspberries
Rutabaga
Spinach
Squash (all varieties)
Strawberries
Swiss chard
Tangerines
Tomatoes
Turnips
Watercress
Watermelon
Zucchini
Protein Sources:
64. Chicken (skinless, breast)

Turkey (skinless, breast)
Fish (salmon, tuna, trout)
Shrimp
Crab
Lobster

Lean cuts of pork (tenderloin, loin chops)
Eggs
Tofu
Tempeh
Cottage cheese (low-fat)
Greek yogurt (unsweetened)
Whole Grains:
77. Quinoa

Brown rice
Oats (steel-cut, rolled)
Bulgur
Buckwheat
Millet
Amaranth
Farro
Barley
Whole grain bread (sprouted, whole wheat)
Whole grain pasta
Wild rice
Nuts and Seeds:
89. Almonds

Walnuts
Pistachios
Cashews
Pecans
Hazelnuts
Macadamia nuts
Chia seeds
Hemp seeds
Sunflower seeds
Pumpkin seeds
Sesame seeds
Dairy and Dairy Alternatives:
101. Greek yogurt (unsweetened)

Cottage cheese (low-fat)

Lean cuts of beef (sirloin, tenderloin)
Skim milk
Soy milk (unsweetened)
Almond milk (unsweetened)
Coconut milk (unsweetened)
Cashew milk (unsweetened)
Healthy Fats:
108. Avocado

Olive oil
Coconut oil
Flaxseed oil
Hempseed oil
Walnut oil
Almond butter
Peanut butter (unsweetened)
Cashew butter (unsweetened)
Herbs and Spices:
117. Basil

Cilantro
Dill
Mint
Oregano
Parsley
Rosemary
Thyme
Turmeric
Cinnamon
Ginger
Garlic powder
Onion powder
Paprika
Chili powder
Cumin
Condiments and Flavorings:
133. Balsamic vinegar

Apple cider vinegar
Dijon mustard

Tamari sauce (low-sodium)
Salsa (unsweetened)
Lemon juice
Lime juice
Stevia (natural sweetener)
Monk fruit extract (natural sweetener)
Coconut aminos
Beverages:
144. Water
Herbal tea (unsweetened)
Green tea (unsweetened)
Black tea (unsweetened)
Coffee (black)
Sparkling water (unsweetened)
Kombucha (unsweetened)
Snacks:
151. Air-popped popcorn
Rice cakes (unsalted, unsweetened)
Veggie sticks (carrots, celery, bell peppers) with hummus
Nuts and seeds (portion-controlled)
Greek yogurt (unsweetened)
Cottage cheese (low-fat)
Hard-boiled eggs
Edamame
Whole grain crackers (portion-controlled)
Seaweed snacks
Frozen Foods:
161. Frozen berries (unsweetened)
Frozen vegetables (broccoli, cauliflower, spinach)
Frozen fish fillets (salmon, tilapia)
Frozen shrimp
Frozen chicken breasts
Frozen fruit bars (unsweetened)
Canned Foods:
167. Canned beans (black beans, kidney beans, chickpeas)
Canned tuna (in water)
Hot sauce (unsweetened)
Canned salmon (in water)
Canned tomatoes (unsweetened)
Canned pumpkin (unsweetened)
Canned coconut milk (unsweetened)
Prepared Foods:
173. Precooked quinoa packets

Precooked brown rice packets
Precooked lentils packets
Precooked chicken breast strips
Precooked shrimp
Precooked tofu
Precooked hard-boiled eggs
Miscellaneous:
180. Nutritional yeast

Hummus
Salsa (unsweetened)
Guacamole
Olives
Pickles
Sauerkraut
Seaweed (nori, wakame)
Unsweetened cocoa powder
Dark chocolate (70% cocoa or higher)
Coconut flakes (unsweetened)
Protein powder (unsweetened)
Unsweetened almond flour
Whole grain flour (whole wheat, spelt, oat)
Unsweetened coconut flour

Grilled Salmon with Asparagus

INGREDIENTS

1. 4 salmon fillets
2. 1 lb asparagus spears
3. 2 tbsp olive oil
4. Salt and pepper to taste
5. Lemon wedges for serving

NUTRITION PER SERVING

Calories: 300

Protein: 25g

Carbohydrates: 5g

Fat: 20g

Fiber: 2g

Prep time: 10 minutes Cook time: 10 minutes

INSTRUCTIONS

Preheat grill to medium-high heat.
Drizzle olive oil over salmon fillets and asparagus. Season with salt and pepper.
Place salmon fillets and asparagus on the grill. Cook salmon for 4-5 minutes per side, or until cooked through. Cook asparagus for 3-4 minutes, or until tender-crisp.
4. Serve grilled salmon and asparagus with lemon wedges.

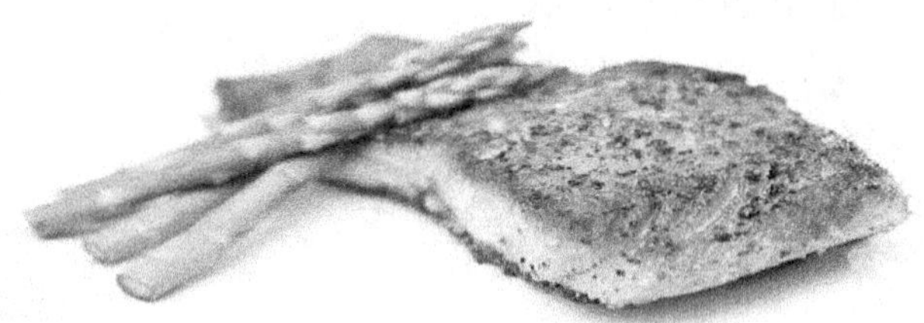

Quinoa Salad with Chickpeas and Roasted Vegetables

INGREDIENTS

1 cup quinoa
1 can chickpeas, drained and rinsed
1 bell pepper, diced
1 zucchini, diced
1 yellow squash, diced
1 red onion, sliced
2 tbsp olive oil
2 tbsp balsamic vinegar
Salt and pepper to taste
Fresh herbs (such as parsley or basil) for garnish

NUTRITION PER SERVING

Calories: 350

Protein: 12g

Carbohydrates: 50g

Fat: 12g

Fiber: 8g

Prep time: 15 minutes Cook time: 25 minutes

INSTRUCTIONS

Preheat oven to 400°F (200°C).
Cook quinoa according to package instructions. Let cool.
In a large bowl, toss chickpeas, bell pepper, zucchini, yellow squash, and red onion with olive oil, balsamic vinegar, salt, and pepper.
Spread vegetables in a single layer on a baking sheet. Roast in the preheated oven for 20-25 minutes, or until tender and slightly caramelized.
In a serving bowl, combine cooked quinoa, roasted vegetables, and chickpeas. Garnish with fresh herbs before serving.

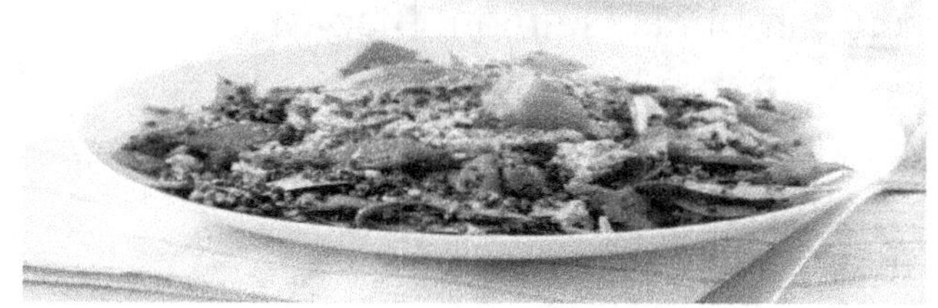

Stir-Fried Tofu with Broccoli and Bell Peppers

INGREDIENTS

1 block firm tofu, pressed and cubed
2 cups broccoli florets
1 bell pepper, sliced
2 cloves garlic, minced
2 tbsp soy sauce
1 tbsp sesame oil
1 tsp cornstarch (optional)
Cooked brown rice for serving

NUTRITION PER SERVING

Calories: 250
Protein: 15g
Carbohydrates: 20g
Fat: 12g
Fiber: 5g
Prep time: 15 minutes Cook time: 15 minutes

INSTRUCTIONS

1. In a large skillet or wok, heat sesame oil over medium heat. Add tofu cubes and cook until golden brown on all sides. Remove tofu from the skillet and set aside.
2. In the same skillet, add broccoli florets, bell pepper slices, and minced garlic. Stir-fry for 5-6 minutes, or until vegetables are tender-crisp.
3. In a small bowl, whisk together soy sauce and cornstarch (if using). Pour sauce over the vegetables and return tofu to the skillet. Stir-fry for an additional 2-3 minutes, or until sauce has thickened.
4. Serve stir-fried tofu and vegetables over cooked brown rice

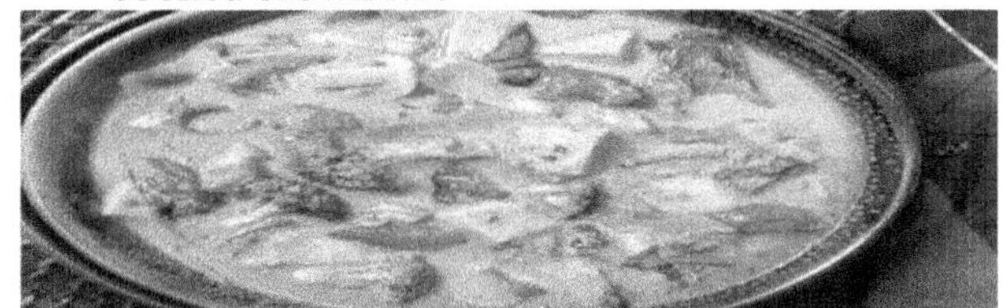

Greek Yogurt Parfait with Berries and Almonds

INGREDIENTS

1 cup Greek yogurt (unsweetened)
1/2 cup mixed berries (such as strawberries, blueberries, raspberries)
1/4 cup almonds, chopped
1 tbsp honey or maple syrup (optional)
1 tsp vanilla extract
1 tbsp chia seeds (optional)

NUTRITION PER SERVING

- o Calories: 200
- o Protein: 15g
- o Carbohydrates: 15g
- o Fat: 10g
- o Fiber: 5g
- Prep time: 5 minutes Cook time: 0 minutes

INSTRUCTIONS

1. In a serving glass or bowl, layer Greek yogurt, mixed berries, and chopped almonds.
2. Drizzle honey or maple syrup over the yogurt and berries if desired. Add a splash of vanilla extract for extra flavor.
3. Top with chia seeds for added texture and nutrition.
4. Repeat layering process until ingredients are used up.
5. Serve immediately or refrigerate for later enjoyment.

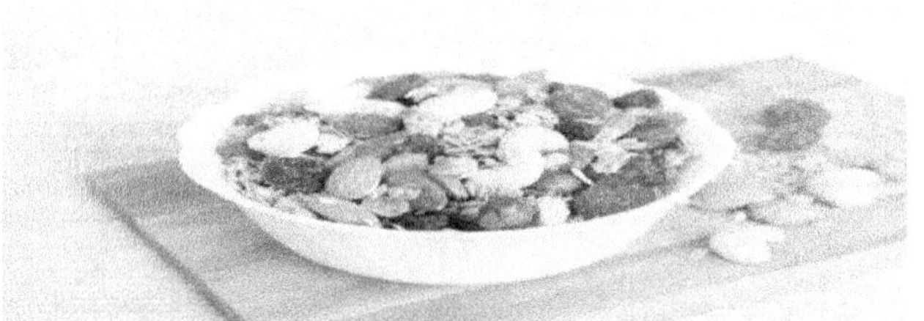

Chicken and Vegetable Stir-Fry with Brown Rice

INGREDIENTS

2 boneless, skinless chicken breasts, thinly sliced
2 cups mixed vegetables(such as bell peppers, broccoli, carrots, snap peas)
2 cloves garlic, minced
2 tbsp soy sauce
1 tbsp hoisin sauce
1 tbsp sesame oil
Cooked brown rice for serving

NUTRITION PER SERVING

Calories: 300

Protein: 25g

Carbohydrates: 30g

Fat: 8g

Fiber: 5g

Prep time: 10 minutes Cook time: 15 minutes

INSTRUCTIONS

1. In a large skillet or wok, heat sesame oil over medium-high heat. Add sliced chicken breasts and minced garlic. Cook until chicken is cooked through, about 5-6 minutes.
2. Add mixed vegetables to the skillet and stir-fry for an additional 4-5 minutes, or until vegetables are tender-crisp.
3. In a small bowl, whisk together soy sauce and hoisin sauce. Pour sauce over chicken and vegetables. Stir to coat evenly.
4. Serve chicken and vegetable stir-fry over cooked brown rice.

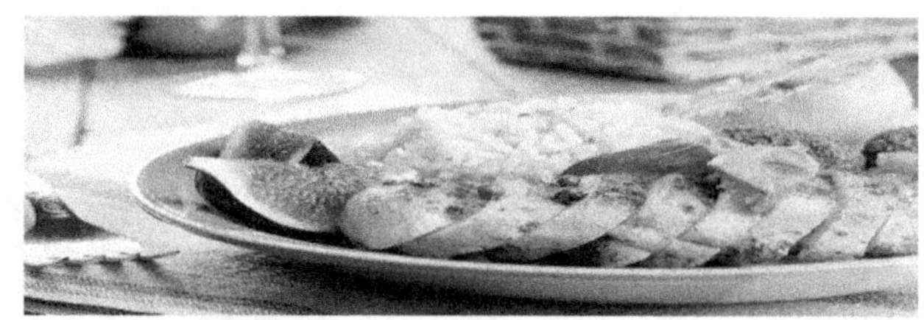

Black Bean and Corn Salad with Avocado

INGREDIENTS

1 can black beans, drained and rinsed
1 cup corn kernels (fresh or frozen)
1 bell pepper, diced
1/2 red onion, diced
1 ripe avocado, diced
2 tbsp lime juice
1 tbsp olive oil
1/4 cup fresh cilantro, chopped
Salt and pepper to taste

NUTRITION PER SERVING

- o   Calories: 250
- o   Protein: 10g
- o   Carbohydrates: 30g
- o   Fat: 12g
- o   Fiber: 10g
- o   Prep time: 10 minutes Cook time: 0 minutes

INSTRUCTIONS

In a large mixing bowl, combine black beans, corn kernels, diced bell pepper, and diced red onion.

Add diced avocado to the bowl and gently toss to combine.

In a small bowl, whisk together lime juice, olive oil, chopped cilantro, salt, and pepper. Pour dressing over the salad and toss to coat evenly.

Serve black bean and corn salad immediately or refrigerate for later enjoyment.

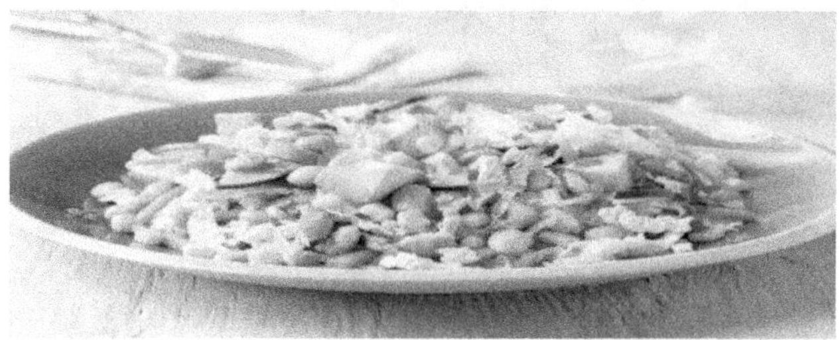

Tuna Salad Lettuce Wraps

INGREDIENTS

2 cans tuna, drained
1/4 cup Greek yogurt (unsweetened)
1 tbsp Dijon mustard
1 stalk celery, diced
1/4 cup red onion, diced
1/4 cup pickles, diced
Salt and pepper to taste
Lettuce leaves for wrapping

NUTRITION PER SERVING

Calories: 200

Protein: 20g

Carbohydrates: 5g

Fat: 10g

Fiber: 2g

Prep time: 10 minutes Cook time: 0 minutes

INSTRUCTIONS

1. In a mixing bowl, combine drained tuna, Greek yogurt, Dijon mustard, diced celery, diced red onion, and diced pickles.
2. Season with salt and pepper to taste. Mix until well combined.
3. Spoon tuna salad mixture onto lettuce leaves and wrap to form lettuce wraps.
4. Serve tuna salad lettuce wraps immediately or refrigerate for later enjoyment.

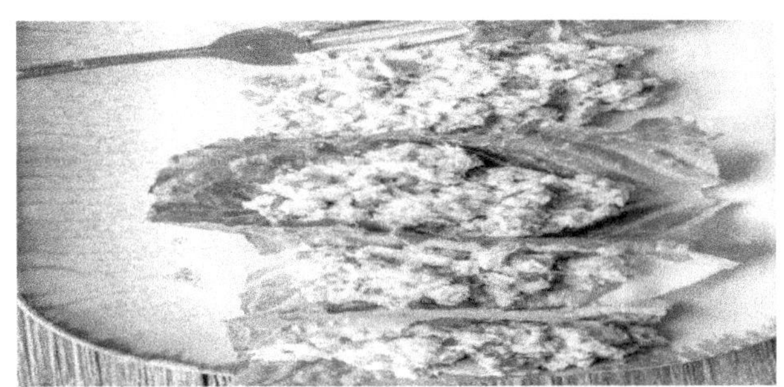

Roasted Vegetable Frittata

INGREDIENTS

6 large eggs
1 cup mixed roasted vegetables (such as bell peppers, zucchini, mushrooms)
1/4 cup shredded cheese (such as cheddar or mozzarella)
2 tbsp milk or unsweetened almond milk
1 tbsp olive oil
Salt and pepper to taste
Fresh herbs for garnish (such as parsley or chives)

NUTRITION PER SERVING

Calories: 250

Protein: 15g

Carbohydrates: 10g

Fat: 15g

Fiber: 3g

Prep time: 10 minutes Cook time: 20 minutes

INSTRUCTIONS

Preheat oven to 375°F (190°C).
In a mixing bowl, whisk together eggs, milk, salt, and pepper until well combined.
Heat olive oil in an oven-safe skillet over medium heat. Add roasted vegetables to the skillet and spread them out evenly.
Pour egg mixture over the vegetables in the skillet. Sprinkle shredded cheese on top.
Transfer the skillet to the preheated oven and bake for 15-20 minutes, or until the frittata is set and golden brown on top.
Remove from the oven and let cool slightly before slicing.
Garnish with fresh herbs before serving.

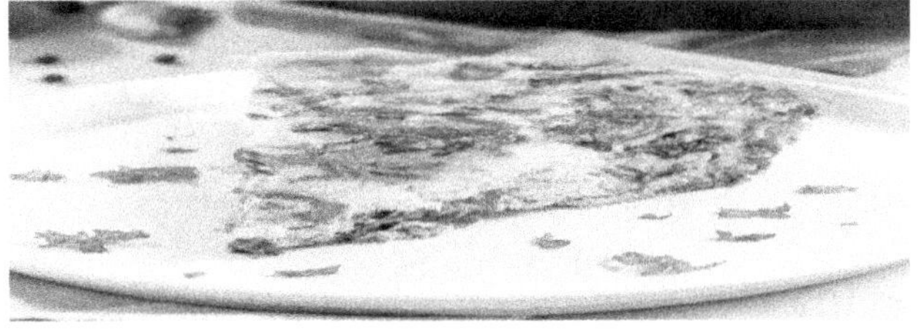

Mediterranean Chickpea Salad

INGREDIENTS

2 cans chickpeas, drained and rinsed
1 cup cherry tomatoes, halved
1/2 cucumber, diced
1/4 cup red onion, diced
1/4 cup Kalamata olives, pitted and halved
1/4 cup crumbled feta cheese
2 tbsp fresh lemon juice
2 tbsp extra virgin olive oil
1 tsp dried oregano
Salt and pepper to taste
Fresh parsley for garnish

NUTRITION PER SERVING

Calories: 300

Protein: 12g

Carbohydrates: 30g

Fat: 15g

Fiber: 8g

Prep time: 10 minutes Cook time: 0 minutes

INSTRUCTIONS

In a large mixing bowl, combine chickpeas, cherry tomatoes, diced cucumber, diced red onion, Kalamata olives, and crumbled feta cheese.

In a small bowl, whisk together lemon juice, olive oil, dried oregano, salt, and pepper to make the dressing.

Pour dressing over the salad ingredients and toss to coat evenly.

Garnish with fresh parsley before serving.

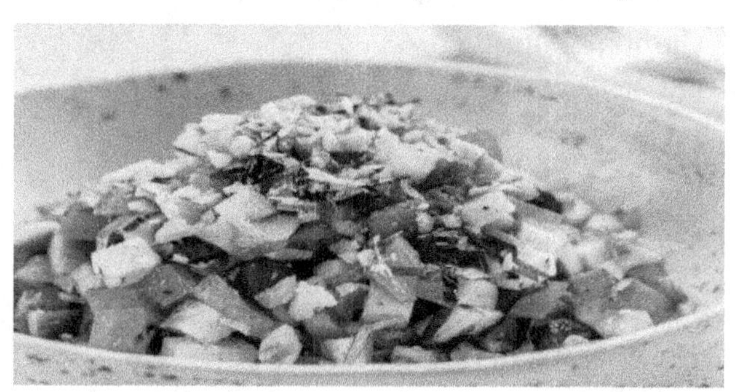

Turkey and Vegetable Lettuce Wraps

INGREDIENTS

1 lb lean ground turkey
1 bell pepper, diced
1/2 onion, diced
2 cloves garlic, minced
1 tsp ground cumin
1 tsp chili powder
1/2 cup salsa (unsweetened)
Salt and pepper to taste
Lettuce leaves for wrapping

NUTRITION PER SERVING

- Calories: 250
- Protein: 25g
- Carbohydrates: 10g
- Fat: 10g
- Fiber: 3g
- Prep time: 10 minutes Cook time: 15 minutes

INSTRUCTIONS

In a large skillet, cook ground turkey over medium heat until browned and cooked through, breaking it up with a spoon as it cooks.

Add diced bell pepper, diced onion, and minced garlic to the skillet. Cook for 3-4 minutes, or until vegetables are tender.

Stir in ground cumin, chili powder, salsa, salt, and pepper. Cook for an additional 2-3 minutes, or until heated through.

Spoon turkey and vegetable mixture onto lettuce leaves and wrap to form lettuce wraps. Serve turkey and vegetable lettuce wraps immediately.

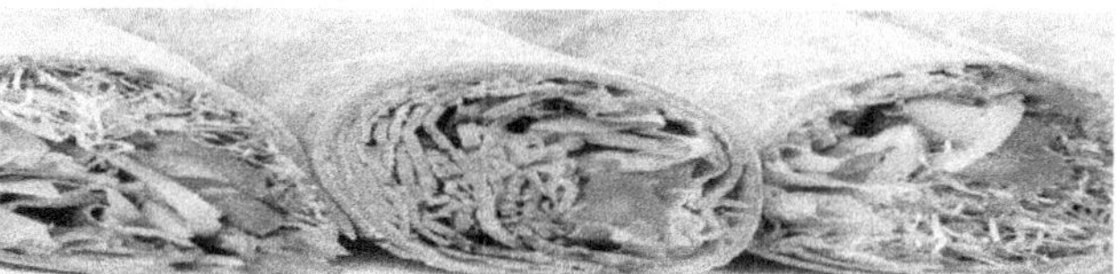

Lemon Herb Grilled Chicken

INGREDIENTS

4 boneless, skinless chicken breasts
Zest and juice of 1 lemon
2 cloves garlic, minced
2 tbsp olive oil
1 tsp dried thyme
1 tsp dried rosemary
Salt and pepper to taste
Lemon wedges for serving

NUTRITION PER SERVING

Calories: 250
Protein: 30g
Carbohydrates: 2g
Fat: 12g
Fiber: 0g
Prep time: 10 minutes (plus marinating time) Cook time: 15 minutes

INSTRUCTIONS

In a small bowl, whisk together lemon zest, lemon juice, minced garlic, olive oil, dried thyme, dried rosemary, salt, and pepper to make the marinade. Place chicken breasts in a shallow dish or resealable plastic bag. Pour the marinade over the chicken, making sure it is evenly coated. Marinate in the refrigerator for at least 30 minutes, or up to 4 hours. Preheat grill to medium-high heat. Remove chicken from marinade and discard any excess marinade. Grill chicken breasts for 6-7 minutes per side, or until cooked through and no longer pink in the center.

Serve grilled lemon herb chicken with lemon wedges for squeezing over the top.

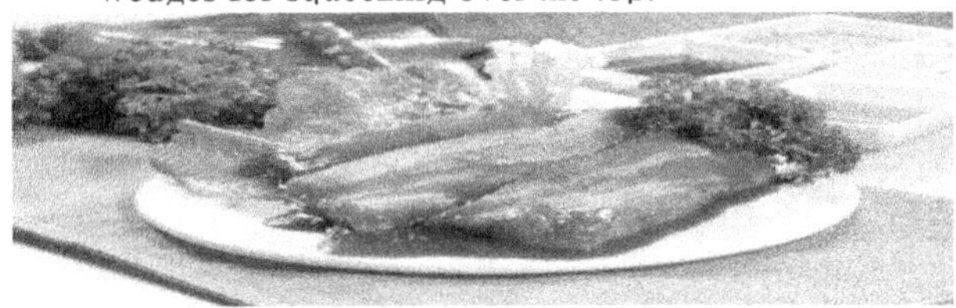

Roasted Vegetable and Quinoa Buddha Bowl

INGREDIENTS

1 cup quinoa
2 cups mixed vegetables (such as sweet potatoes, Brussels sprouts, carrots)
2 tbsp olive oil
1 tsp smoked paprika
1 tsp garlic powder
Salt and pepper to taste
1/4 cup hummus
1/4 cup tahini dressing (store-bought or homemade)

NUTRITION PER SERVING

o   Calories: 350
o   Protein: 10g
o   Carbohydrates: 40g
o   Fat: 15g
o   Fiber: 8g
o   Prep time: 15 minutes
    Cook time: 25 minutes

INSTRUCTIONS

Preheat oven to 400°F (200°C).
Cook quinoa according to package instructions. Set aside.
In a large mixing bowl, toss mixed vegetables with olive oil, smoked paprika, garlic powder, salt, and pepper until evenly coated.
Spread seasoned vegetables in a single layer on a baking sheet. Roast in the preheated oven for 20-25 minutes, or until tender and caramelized.
Divide cooked quinoa among serving bowls. Top with roasted vegetables, hummus, and a drizzle of tahini dressing.
Serve roasted vegetable and quinoa Buddha bowls immediately.

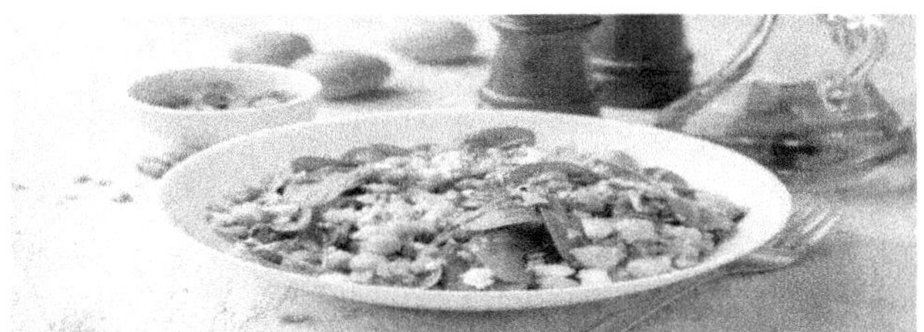

Spinach and Mushroom Omelette

INGREDIENTS

3 large eggs
1 cup fresh spinach leaves
1/2 cup sliced mushrooms
2 tbsp shredded cheese (such as mozzarella or feta)
1 tsp olive oil
Salt and pepper to taste

NUTRITION PER SERVING

Calories: 250

Protein: 20g

Carbohydrates: 3g

Fat: 15g

Fiber: 1g

Prep time: 5 minutes Cook time: 10 minutes

INSTRUCTIONS

In a small mixing bowl, whisk together eggs, salt, and pepper until well combined.

Heat olive oil in a non-stick skillet over medium heat. Add spinach leaves and sliced mushrooms to the skillet. Cook until spinach is wilted and mushrooms are tender.

Pour whisked eggs evenly over the cooked spinach and mushrooms. Cook for 2-3 minutes, or until the edges of the omelette begin to set.

Sprinkle shredded cheese over one half of the omelette. Fold the other half over the cheese to form a half-moon shape.

Cook for an additional 1-2 minutes, or until the cheese is melted and the omelette is cooked through.

Serve spinach and mushroom omelette hot.

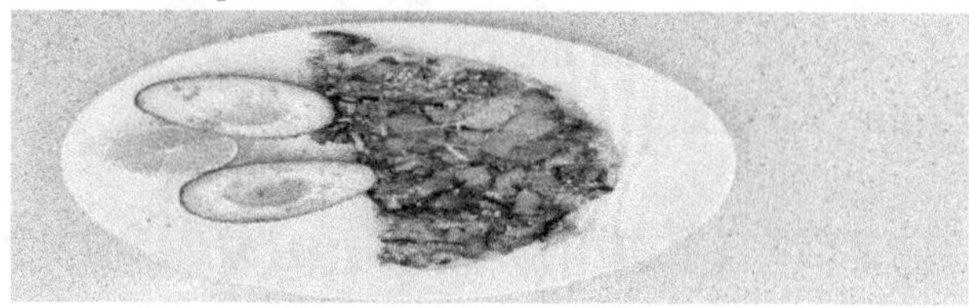

Lentil and Vegetable Soup

INGREDIENTS

1 cup dried green lentils, rinsed
4 cups vegetable broth
2 cups mixed vegetables (such as carrots, celery, bell peppers)
1 onion, diced
2 cloves garlic, minced
1 tsp dried thyme
1 tsp dried oregano
Salt and pepper to taste
Fresh parsley for garnish

NUTRITION PER SERVING

- Calories: 200
- Protein: 12g
- Carbohydrates: 30g
- Fat: 2g
- Fiber: 10g
- Prep time: 10 minutes Cook time: 40 minutes

INSTRUCTIONS

In a large pot, combine dried lentils, vegetable broth, diced onion, minced garlic, dried thyme, dried oregano, salt, and pepper.

Bring the soup to a boil over medium-high heat. Reduce heat to low, cover, and simmer for 20-25 minutes, or until lentils are tender.

Add mixed vegetables to the pot and simmer for an additional 10-15 minutes, or until vegetables are tender.

Adjust seasoning with salt and pepper if needed.

Serve lentil and vegetable soup hot, garnished with fresh parsley.

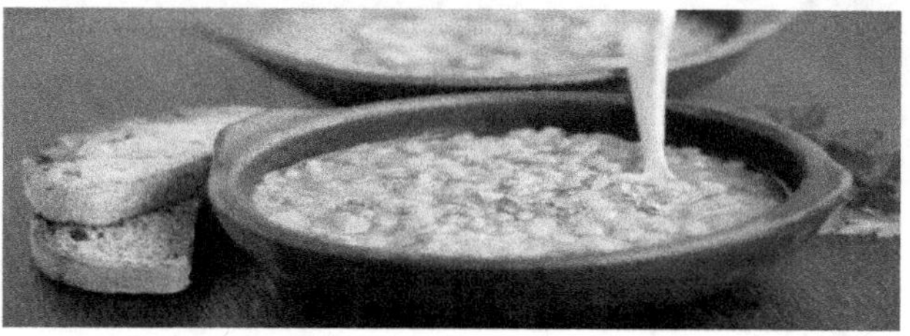

Mango Chicken Salad

INGREDIENTS

2 boneless, skinless chicken breasts
1 ripe mango, diced
1/2 cucumber, diced
1/4 cup red onion, diced
1/4 cup fresh cilantro, chopped
Juice of 1 lime
2 tbsp olive oil
Salt and pepper to taste
Mixed greens for serving

NUTRITION PER SERVING

- Calories: 300
- Protein: 25g
- Carbohydrates: 20g
- Fat: 15g
- Fiber: 5g
- Prep time: 10 minutes Cook time: 15 minutes

INSTRUCTIONS

Season chicken breasts with salt and pepper. Grill or pan-sear until cooked through, about 6-7 minutes per side. Let cool slightly, then slice into strips.

In a large mixing bowl, combine diced mango, diced cucumber, diced red onion, chopped cilantro, lime juice, and olive oil. Toss to combine.

Add sliced chicken to the bowl and gently toss to coat with the mango salsa mixture.

Serve mango chicken salad over a bed of mixed greens.

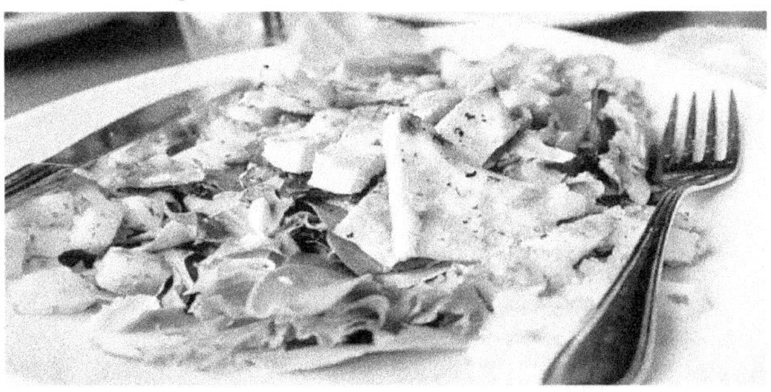

Turkey and Black Bean Chili

INGREDIENTS

1 lb lean ground turkey
1 can black beans, drained and rinsed
1 can diced tomatoes
1 bell pepper, diced
1 onion, diced
2 cloves garlic, minced
1 tbsp chili powder
1 tsp ground cumin
1/2 tsp smoked paprika
Salt and pepper to taste
Fresh cilantro for garnish
Greek yogurt for serving (optional)

NUTRITION PER SERVING

- Calories: 300
- Protein: 25g
- Carbohydrates: 30g
- Fat: 10g
- Fiber: 10g
- Prep time: 10 minutes Cook time: 30 minutes

INSTRUCTIONS

In a large pot, cook ground turkey over medium heat until browned and cooked through. Drain any excess fat.

Add diced onion, diced bell pepper, and minced garlic to the pot. Cook for 3-4 minutes, or until vegetables are softened.

Stir in chili powder, ground cumin, smoked paprika, salt, and pepper. Cook for an additional 1-2 minutes, or until fragrant.

Add black beans and diced tomatoes to the pot. Bring the chili to a simmer and let cook for 20-25 minutes, stirring occasionally.

Adjust seasoning with salt and pepper if needed. Serve turkey and black bean chili hot, garnished with fresh cilantro. Serve with a dollop of Greek yogurt if desired.

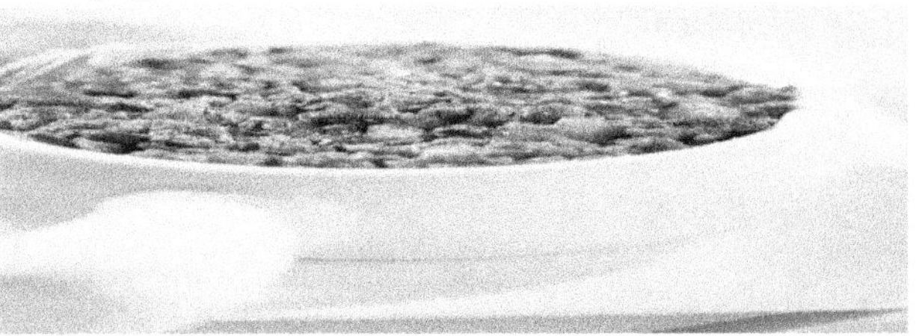

Sweet Potato and Black Bean Tacos

INGREDIENTS

2 large sweet potatoes, peeled and diced
1 can black beans, drained and rinsed
1 bell pepper, diced
1/2 onion, diced
2 cloves garlic, minced
1 tbsp olive oil
1 tsp chili powder
1/2 tsp ground cumin
Salt and pepper to taste
Corn tortillas for serving
Avocado slices for garnish
Fresh cilantro for garnish

NUTRITION PER SERVING

- Calories: 250
- Protein: 8g
- Carbohydrates: 35g
- Fat: 10g
- Fiber: 8g
- Prep time: 15 minutes Cook time: 25 minutes

INSTRUCTIONS

Preheat oven to 400°F (200°C).

Toss diced sweet potatoes with olive oil, chili powder, ground cumin, salt, and pepper until evenly coated.

Spread seasoned sweet potatoes in a single layer on a baking sheet. Roast in the preheated oven for 20-25 minutes, or until tender and caramelized.

In a skillet, heat olive oil over medium heat. Add diced bell pepper, diced onion, and minced garlic. Cook for 3-4 minutes, or until vegetables are softened.

Add black beans to the skillet and cook for an additional 2-3 minutes, or until heated through.

Warm corn tortillas in a dry skillet or microwave.

Assemble tacos by filling each tortilla with roasted sweet potatoes, black bean mixture, avocado slices, and fresh cilantro.

Serve sweet potato and black bean tacos immediately.

Greek Chicken Skewers with Tzatziki Sauce

INGREDIENTS

1 lb chicken breast, cut into cubes
1 bell pepper, cut into chunks
1 red onion, cut into chunks
1/4 cup olive oil
2 cloves garlic, minced
1 tsp dried oregano
1 tsp dried thyme
Salt and pepper to taste
Wooden skewers, soaked in water for 30 minutes
Tzatziki sauce for serving

NUTRITION PER SERVING

- Calories: 300
- Protein: 25g
- Carbohydrates: 10g
- Fat: 15g
- Fiber: 2g
- Prep time: 15 minutes (plus marinating time) Cook time: 10 minutes

INSTRUCTIONS

In a mixing bowl, combine olive oil, minced garlic, dried oregano, dried thyme, salt, and pepper.

Add chicken breast cubes to the bowl and toss to coat evenly. Cover and marinate in the refrigerator for at least 30 minutes, or up to 4 hours.

Preheat grill or grill pan to medium-high heat.

Thread marinated chicken cubes, bell pepper chunks, and red onion chunks onto wooden skewers.

Grill chicken skewers for 4-5 minutes per side, or until chicken is cooked through and vegetables are tender.

Serve Greek chicken skewers hot, with tzatziki sauce for dipping.

Mushroom and Spinach Stuffed Chicken Breast

INGREDIENTS

4 boneless, skinless chicken breasts
1 cup chopped mushrooms
2 cups fresh spinach leaves
1/4 cup shredded mozzarella cheese
2 cloves garlic, minced
2 tbsp olive oil
Salt and pepper to taste

NUTRITION PER SERVING

- Calories: 300
- Protein: 30g
- Carbohydrates: 5g
- Fat: 15g
- Fiber: 2g
- Prep time: 15 minutes Cook time: 30 minutes

INSTRUCTIONS

Preheat oven to 375°F (190°C).

In a skillet, heat olive oil over medium heat. Add chopped mushrooms and minced garlic. Cook for 5-6 minutes, or until mushrooms are tender and golden brown. Add spinach leaves to the skillet and cook for an additional 2-3 minutes, or until wilted. Season with salt and pepper.

Using a sharp knife, make a horizontal slit along the side of each chicken breast to create a pocket.

Stuff each chicken breast with the mushroom and spinach mixture, then sprinkle shredded mozzarella cheese on top.

Secure the openings of the chicken breasts with toothpicks to keep the stuffing in place.

Place stuffed chicken breasts in a baking dish and drizzle with a little olive oil.

Bake in the preheated oven for 25-30 minutes, or until chicken is cooked through and cheese is melted and bubbly.

Serve mushroom and spinach stuffed chicken breasts hot.

Salmon and Asparagus Sheet Pan Dinner

INGREDIENTS

4 salmon fillets
1 lb asparagus spears, trimmed
2 tbsp olive oil
2 cloves garlic, minced
1 tsp lemon zest
Salt and pepper to taste
Lemon wedges for serving

NUTRITION PER SERVING

Calories: 350

Protein: 30g

Carbohydrates: 5g

Fat: 20g

Fiber: 2g

- Prep time: 10 minutes Cook time: 15 minutes

INSTRUCTIONS

Preheat oven to 400°F (200°C).

Place salmon fillets and asparagus spears on a large baking sheet lined with parchment paper.

In a small bowl, whisk together olive oil, minced garlic, lemon zest, salt, and pepper. Drizzle the mixture over the salmon and asparagus, tossing to coat evenly.

Arrange salmon fillets skin-side down on the baking sheet, leaving space between each fillet. Place asparagus spears alongside the salmon.

Bake in the preheated oven for 12-15 minutes, or until salmon is cooked through and flakes easily with a fork, and asparagus is tender-crisp.

Serve salmon and asparagus sheet pan dinner hot, with lemon wedges for squeezing over the top.

Vegetable and Lentil Curry

INGREDIENTS

1 cup dried lentils, rinsed
2 cups vegetable broth
1 onion, diced
2 cloves garlic, minced
1 bell pepper, diced
1 zucchini, diced
1 carrot, diced
1 cup diced tomatoes
1 can coconut milk
2 tbsp curry powder
1 tsp ground turmeric
Salt and pepper to taste
Fresh cilantro for garnish
Cooked rice for serving

NUTRITION PER SERVING

- Calories: 300
- Protein: 15g
- Carbohydrates: 30g
- Fat: 15g
- Fiber: 10g
- Prep time: 10 minutes Cook time: 30 minutes

INSTRUCTIONS

In a large pot, combine dried lentils, vegetable broth, diced onion, minced garlic, diced bell pepper, diced zucchini, diced carrot, diced tomatoes, coconut milk, curry powder, ground turmeric, salt, and pepper.

Bring the curry to a boil over medium-high heat. Reduce heat to low, cover, and simmer for 20-25 minutes, or until lentils are tender and the curry has thickened.

Adjust seasoning with salt and pepper if needed.

Serve vegetable and lentil curry hot, garnished with fresh cilantro. Serve over cooked rice.

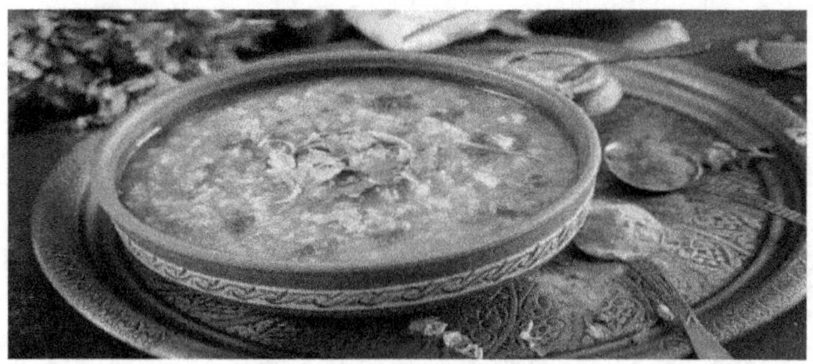

Cauliflower Rice Stir-Fry

INGREDIENTS

1 head cauliflower, riced
2 cups mixed vegetables (such as bell peppers, broccoli, snap peas)
2 cloves garlic, minced
2 tbsp soy sauce
1 tbsp sesame oil
1 tsp grated ginger
Salt and pepper to taste
Cooked protein of choice (such as tofu, chicken, shrimp) (optional)

NUTRITION PER SERVING

- Calories: 150
- Protein: 5g
- Carbohydrates: 15g
- Fat: 8g
- Fiber: 8g
- Prep time: 10 minutes Cook time: 10 minutes

INSTRUCTIONS

- Heat sesame oil in a large skillet or wok over medium-high heat. Add minced garlic and grated ginger. Cook for 1-2 minutes, or until fragrant.
- Add mixed vegetables to the skillet and stir-fry for 3-4 minutes, or until tender-crisp.
- Add riced cauliflower to the skillet and stir-fry for an additional 2-3 minutes, or until cauliflower is cooked through.
- Stir in soy sauce and cooked protein of choice (if using). Cook for an additional 1-2 minutes, or until heated through.
- Adjust seasoning with salt and pepper if needed.
- Serve cauliflower rice stir-fry hot.

Baked Cod with Lemon and Herbs

INGREDIENTS

- 4 cod fillets
- Zest and juice of 1 lemon
- 2 tbsp chopped fresh herbs (such as parsley, dill, or thyme)
- 2 cloves garlic, minced
- 2 tbsp olive oil
- Salt and pepper to taste
- Lemon slices for serving

NUTRITION PER SERVING

- Calories: 200
- Protein: 25g
- Carbohydrates: 2g
- Fat: 10g
- Fiber: 1g
- Prep time: 10 minutes Cook time: 15 minutes

INSTRUCTIONS

- Preheat oven to 400°F (200°C).
- In a small bowl, combine lemon zest, chopped fresh herbs, minced garlic, olive oil, salt, and pepper to make the marinade.
- Place cod fillets in a baking dish. Pour the marinade over the cod, making sure it is evenly coated.
- Bake in the preheated oven for 12-15 minutes, or until cod is cooked through and flakes easily with a fork.
- Serve baked cod with lemon slices for squeezing over the top.

Caprese Stuffed Chicken Breast

INGREDIENTS

- 4 boneless, skinless chicken breasts
- 1 cup cherry tomatoes, halved
- 1/2 cup fresh mozzarella cheese, diced
- 1/4 cup fresh basil leaves, chopped
- 2 cloves garlic, minced
- 2 tbsp balsamic vinegar
- 2 tbsp olive oil
- Salt and pepper to taste

NUTRITION PER SERVING

- Calories: 250
- Protein: 30g
- Carbohydrates: 5g
- Fat: 12g
- Fiber: 1g
- Prep time: 15 minutes Cook time: 30 minutes

INSTRUCTIONS

Preheat oven to 375°F (190°C).

In a mixing bowl, combine halved cherry tomatoes, diced fresh mozzarella cheese, chopped fresh basil leaves, minced garlic, balsamic vinegar, olive oil, salt, and pepper. Toss to combine.

Using a sharp knife, make a horizontal slit along the side of each chicken breast to create a pocket.

Stuff each chicken breast with the caprese mixture.

Secure the openings of the chicken breasts with toothpicks to keep the stuffing in place.

Place stuffed chicken breasts in a baking dish.

Bake in the preheated oven for 25-30 minutes, or until chicken is cooked through.

Serve caprese stuffed chicken breast hot.

Broccoli and Cheddar Quiche

INGREDIENTS

- 1 pre-made pie crust
- 4 large eggs
- 1 cup milk or unsweetened almond milk
- 2 cups chopped broccoli florets
- 1 cup shredded cheddar cheese
- 1/2 onion, diced
- 2 cloves garlic, minced
- Salt and pepper to taste

NUTRITION PER SERVING

- Calories: 300
- Protein: 15g
- Carbohydrates: 20g
- Fat: 18g
- Fiber: 2g
- Prep time: 15 minutes Cook time: 40 minutes

INSTRUCTIONS

- Preheat oven to 375°F (190°C).
- Roll out pre-made pie crust and place it in a pie dish.
- In a mixing bowl, whisk together eggs, milk, salt, and pepper until well combined.
- Spread chopped broccoli florets, diced onion, minced garlic, and shredded cheddar cheese evenly in the pie crust.
- Pour egg mixture over the broccoli, onion, garlic, and cheese in the pie crust.
- Bake in the preheated oven for 35-40 minutes, or until the quiche is set and golden brown on top.
- Let cool slightly before slicing and serving.

Zucchini Noodles with Pesto and Cherry Tomatoes

INGREDIENTS

- 4 medium zucchini, spiralized
- 1 cup cherry tomatoes, halved
- 1/4 cup basil pesto
- 2 tbsp grated Parmesan cheese
- Salt and pepper to taste

NUTRITION PER SERVING

- Calories: 200
- Protein: 5g
- Carbohydrates: 10g
- Fat: 15g
- Fiber: 3g
- Prep time: 10 minutes Cook time: 10 minutes

INSTRUCTIONS

- In a large skillet, heat olive oil over medium heat. Add spiralized zucchini noodles to the skillet and cook for 2-3 minutes, or until just tender.
- Add halved cherry tomatoes to the skillet and cook for an additional 1-2 minutes, or until tomatoes are slightly softened.
- Remove skillet from heat and stir in basil pesto until zucchini noodles and cherry tomatoes are evenly coated.
- Season with salt and pepper to taste.
- Serve zucchini noodles with pesto and cherry tomatoes hot, garnished with grated Parmesan cheese.

Stuffed Bell Peppers with Quinoa and Black Beans

INGREDIENTS

- 4 large bell peppers
- 1 cup cooked quinoa
- 1 can black beans, drained and rinsed
- 1 cup diced tomatoes
- 1/2 cup diced onion
- 2 cloves garlic, minced
- 1 tsp ground cumin
- 1 tsp chili powder
- Salt and pepper to taste
- Shredded cheese for topping (optional)
- Fresh cilantro for garnish

NUTRITION PER SERVING

- Calories: 250
- Protein: 10g
- Carbohydrates: 30g
- Fat: 5g
- Fiber: 8g
- Prep time: 15 minutes
  Cook time: 30 minutes

INSTRUCTIONS

- Preheat oven to 375°F (190°C).
- Cut the tops off the bell peppers and remove the seeds and membranes. Place the hollowed-out peppers in a baking dish.
- In a large mixing bowl, combine cooked quinoa, black beans, diced tomatoes, diced onion, minced garlic, ground cumin, chili powder, salt, and pepper.
- Spoon the quinoa and black bean mixture evenly into the bell peppers.
- Cover the baking dish with aluminum foil and bake in the preheated oven for 25-30 minutes, or until the bell peppers are tender.
- If using shredded cheese, remove the foil from the baking dish and sprinkle cheese over the stuffed bell peppers. Return to the oven and bake for an additional 5 minutes, or until the cheese is melted and bubbly.
- Garnish stuffed bell peppers with fresh cilantro before serving.

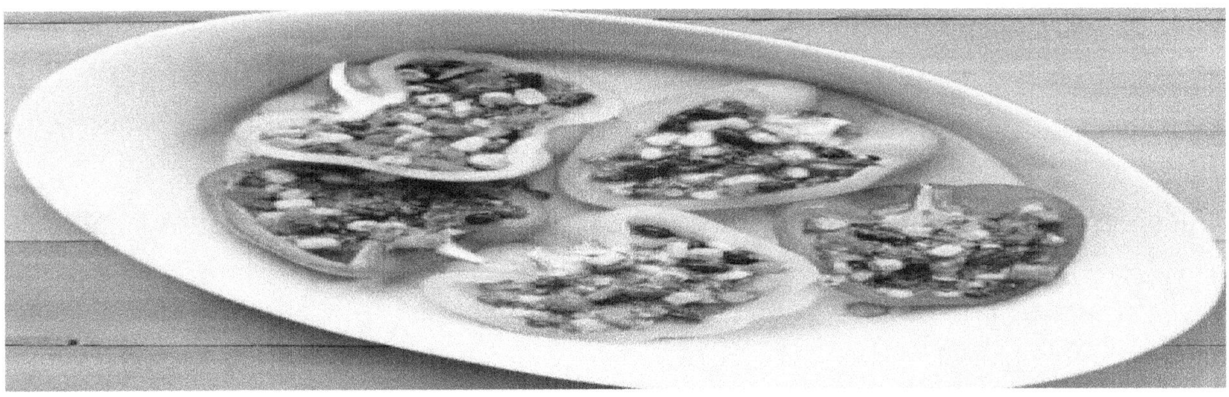

Conclusion

As we explore the wide world of foods that are suitable for diabetics and prepare delicious meals, we have had a life-changing experience. We have explored the world of nutrient-rich foods in great detail, examined the science behind glycemic load and glycemic index, and refined our meal-planning techniques for the best possible control of diabetes via the pages of this thorough book.

As we come to the end of our culinary tour, it is important to consider the significant influence that eating may have on our overall health and well-being. Beyond just sating our hunger, the decisions we make in the kitchen can impact every aspect of our lives, from blood sugar levels to long-term health consequences.

We've opened the door to better blood sugar regulation and enhanced general health by adopting a diet high in foods with low glycemic load. By choosing foods carefully and preparing meals with consideration, we have discovered how to feed our bodies in ways that support resilience and vitality.

But this is not where our trip ends. Equipped with the information and abilities found inside these pages, we can now go forward with our investigation of wholesome, diabetes-friendly food. Let's take a thoughtful and imaginative approach to every meal, turning it from a chore to a celebration of life and health.

As you go into the world of food outside of these pages, never forget that you can improve your health. You have the chance to provide your body with the sustenance it needs with every item you choose and every meal you cook, laying the groundwork for a healthy and happy life.

I hope that this book will be a source of inspiration for you as you continue on your path to the best possible health and well-being. Accept the myriad of tastes and sensations that nature provides, and enjoy every second that you spend providing nourishment for your body and spirit.

Cheers to a brighter future full of tasty, diabetes-friendly food and healthy health.

Appendices

ADDITIONAL RESOURCES FOR FURTHER READING

Day	Breakfast	Lunch	Dinner
Day 1	Scrambled eggs	Grilled chicken salad	Baked salmon with vegetables

| **Day 2** | Greek yogurt with berries | Turkey and vegetable stir-fry | Cauliflower rice with tofu |

| **Day 3** | Oatmeal with nuts | Lentil soup | Zucchini noodles with pesto |

| **Day 4** | Whole grain toast with avocado | Quinoa salad | Beef stir-fry with broccoli |

| **Day 5** | Smoothie | Chicken Caesar salad | Stuffed bell peppers |

| **Day 6** | Cottage cheese with fruit | Vegetable omelette | Baked cod with asparagus |

| **Day 7** | Chia pudding | Tuna salad sandwich | Eggplant parmesan |

| **Day 8** | Breakfast burrito | Chickpea salad | Grilled shrimp skewers |

| **Day 9** | Pancakes with sugar-free syrup | Spinach and mushroom quiche | Teriyaki tofu with rice |

| **Day 10** | Breakfast muffins | Caprese stuffed chicken breast | Vegetable curry |

Day 11	Avocado toast with sauce	Black bean soup	Spaghetti squash
Day 12	Fruit salad	Quinoa and black bean tacos	Chicken and vegetable stir-fry
Day 13	Smoothie bowl	Greek salad	Baked turkey meatballs
Day 14	Scrambled tofu	Lentil and vegetable stew	Grilled vegetable skewers
Day 15	Yogurt parfait	Turkey and avocado wrap	Salmon with quinoa salad
Day 16	Breakfast burrito	Chicken and vegetable stir-fry	Stuffed bell peppers
Day 17	Oatmeal with fresh fruit	Lentil soup	Eggplant parmesan
Day 18	Greek yogurt with nuts	Quinoa salad	Baked cod with asparagus
Day 19	Whole grain toast with avocado	Chickpea salad	Teriyaki tofu with rice
Day 20	Smoothie	Caprese stuffed chicken breast	Vegetable curry
Day 21	Cottage cheese with berries	Black bean soup	Spaghetti squash with sauce
Day 22	Chia pudding	Quinoa and black bean tacos	Chicken and vegetable stir-fry

Day 23	Pancakes with sugar-free syrup	Greek salad	Grilled vegetable skewers
Day 24	Breakfast muffins	Lentil and vegetable stew	Baked turkey meatballs
Day 25	Avocado toast	Turkey and avocado wrap	Salmon with quinoa salad
Day 26	Fruit salad	Chicken and vegetable stir-fry	Stuffed bell peppers
Day 27	Smoothie bowl	Quinoa salad	Eggplant parmesan
Day 28	Scrambled tofu	Chickpea salad	Baked cod with asparagus
Day 29	Yogurt parfait	Caprese stuffed chicken breast	Teriyaki tofu with rice
Day 30	Breakfast burrito	Black bean soup	Vegetable curry

Date........./....../.........

ingredient

note

Description

prep time: cook time:

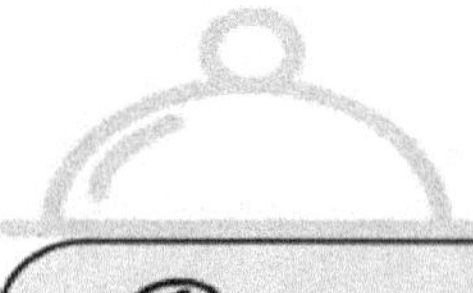

Date.........,/....../.........

Recipe Title:

ingredient

note

Description

prep time: cook time:

Date.........,/....../.........

Recipe Title:

ingredient

note

Description

prep time: cook time:

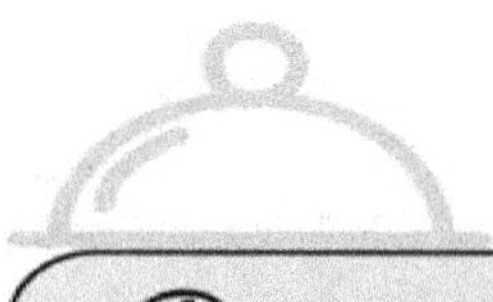

Recipe Title:

ingredient

note

Description

prep time: cook time:

weekly Meal planner

For the week of : ___________________________

Monday

B

L

S

D

Tuesday

B

L

S

D

Wednessday

B

L

S

D

Thursday

B

L

S

D

Friday

B

L

S

D

Saturday

B

L

S

D

sunday

B

L

S

D

shopping list

BLOOD SUGAR LONG TRACKER

STARTING POINT

ENDING

NOTE

weekly Meal planner

For the week of : _______________________________

Monday

B	
L	
S	
D	

Tuesday

B	
L	
S	
D	

Wednessday

B	
L	
S	
D	

Thursday

B	
L	
S	
D	

Friday

B	
L	
S	
D	

Saturday

B	
L	
S	
D	

sunday

B	
L	
S	
D	

shopping list

BLOOD SUGAR LONG TRACKER

STARTING POINT

ENDING

NOTE

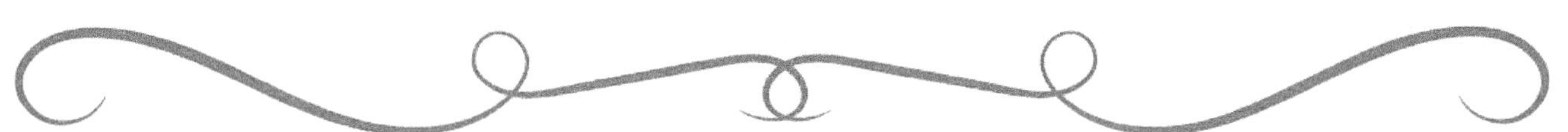

Acknowledgments

We extend our heartfelt gratitude to the healthcare professionals, researchers, and individuals living with diabetes who have contributed their expertise, insights, and experiences to the creation of this book. Your dedication to advancing the field of diabetes management and improving the lives of others is truly commendable. We also express our appreciation to our families, friends, and colleagues for their unwavering support and encouragement throughout this endeavor. Together, we are united in our commitment to empowering individuals with the knowledge and tools needed to thrive in the face of diabetes.

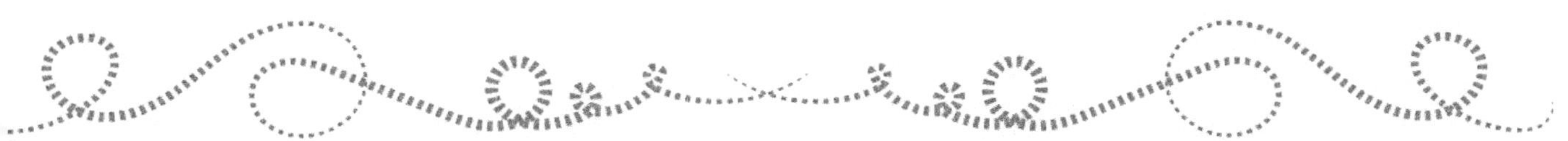